Invisible Illnesses: An A – Z of Hidden Conditions and Rare Diseases

Paul Andrew Smith

Copyright © 2020 by Paul Andrew Smith

The right of Paul Andrew Smith to be identified as the author of this book has been asserted by him in accordance with the Copyright, Designs and Patents Act 1988.
All rights reserved. No part of this publication may be reproduced, distributed, or transmitted in any form or by any means, including photocopying, recording, or other electronic or mechanical methods, without the prior written permission of the publisher, except in the case of brief quotations embodied in critical reviews and certain other non-commercial uses permitted by copyright law. For permission requests, write to the copyright owner or publisher.

Acknowledgements

I would like to thank Annabel Venn for bringing this book to life.

CONTENTS

INTRODUCTION 1

Addiction 3

Addison's Disease 5

Allergies 7

Alzheimer's Disease 9

Ankylosing Spondylitis 11

Anxiety Disorders 13

Arachnoiditis 15

Arthritis 17

Asperger's Syndrome 19

Asthma 21

Attention Deficit Hyperactivity Disorder (ADHD) 23

Autism 25

Benign Prostatic Hyperplasia 27

Bipolar Disorder 29

Body Dysmorphic Disorder 31

Borderline Personality Disorder 33

Brittle Bone Disease 35

Bronchiectasis 37

Cancer 39

Charcot-Marie-Tooth Disease 41

Chronic Fatigue Syndrome 43

Chronic Obstructive Pulmonary Disease 45

Chronic Pain Syndrome 47

Chronic Exertional Compartment Syndrome 49

Coeliac Disease 51

Complex Regional Pain Syndrome 53

Crohn's Disease 55

Cystic Fibrosis 57

Depression 59

Dermatomyositis 61

Diabetes 63

Dissociation and Dissociative Disorders 65

Dyslexia 67

Dyspraxia 69

Dystonia 71

Eating Disorders 73

Ehlers-Danlos Syndrome 75

Encephalitis 77

Endometriosis	79
Epilepsy	81
Fetal Alcohol Spectrum Disorders	83
Fibromyalgia	85
Food Allergies	87
Friedreich's Ataxia	89
Hereditary Fructose Intolerance	91
Fructose Malabsorption	93
Hashimoto's Thyroiditis	95
HIV and AIDS	97
Hyperhidrosis	99
Hypoglycaemia	101
Inclusion Body Myositis	103
Interstitial Cystitis	105
Irritable Bowel Syndrome	107
Kennedy's Disease	109
Lactose Intolerance	111
Lupus	113
Lyme Disease	115
Metabolic Syndrome	117

Migraines	119
Multiple Chemical Sensitivity	121
Multiple Sclerosis	123
Multiple System Atrophy	125
Myasthenia Gravis	127
Narcolepsy	129
Osteoporosis	131
Overactive Thyroid Gland	133
Personality Disorders	135
Phobias	137
Polycystic Ovary Syndrome	139
Polymyositis	141
Post-Traumatic Stress Disorder	143
Primary Immunodeficiency Disorders	145
Prosopagnosia	147
Proteus Syndrome	149
Pulmonary Fibrosis	151
Pulmonary Hypertension	153
Raynaud's	155
Restless Legs Syndrome	157

Schizophrenia 159

Schnitzler Syndrome 161

Scleroderma 163

Seasonal Affective Disorder 165

Sjögren's Syndrome 167

Sleep Disorders 169

Spinal Muscular Atrophy 171

Syringomyelia 173

Tardive Dyskinesia 175

Temporomandibular Joint Disorder 177

Tourette's Syndrome 179

Transverse Myelitis 181

Trigeminal Neuralgia 183

Ulcerative Colitis 185

Vascular Dementia 187

SUMMARY 189

INTRODUCTION

Millions of people in the world are living with hidden illnesses, many with no visible symptoms at all. Due to their unseen nature, and some of them sharing similar or even the same symptoms, many of the disorders are hard to identify and can often go undiagnosed or misdiagnosed for months or years. Some conditions do not qualify as a 'disability' yet can be debilitating to the individual, with symptoms having a negative impact on education, employment or social life. Symptoms can flare up unexpectedly or in response to certain triggers and can be difficult to manage on a daily basis.

For people living with these conditions, sometimes there is also an internal battle to overcome – fearful of making their illness known due to potential discrimination or stigmatisation, largely the result of a lack of education about the condition. With society and workplaces slowly changing, adapting and becoming more accepting, it presents new opportunities for people to no longer suffer in silence. Whilst this book is designed to be a brief snapshot into some of the most unknown and misunderstood conditions, further research and information can be sourced from your doctor or online. Much of the research for this book was sourced directly from the National Health Service (NHS) and other reputable medical sources. If you or someone you know has an invisible illness, then it's important to remember that you or they are not alone. In the majority of cases, specialist charitable organisations exist to help those who have been diagnosed with medical conditions.

Addiction

Similar but not identical to a dependency, Addiction is an uncontrollable obsession over something that can have a damaging or adverse impact. Whilst there is evidence that addictive behaviour can be genetic, the probability of developing an addiction is increased by environmental and social factors, largely stressful life events. Biological factors also play a part, including chemical imbalances or malfunctions of specific areas of the brain. As a form of coping mechanism, addictions are also intrinsically connected to other mental health conditions. Many addictions are never formally identified or diagnosed, but it is believed that around a third of adults in the UK could be addicted to something.

The classic, well-recognised addictions are those of alcohol, drugs or solvents, nicotine and gambling. However, it is possible for an individual to become addicted to anything that provides a seemingly positive impact on their mental state; work, food (including sugar, chocolate or caffeine), exercise, technology (or the Internet or social media) or shopping. Indications of an addiction are an intense desire for a behaviour or substance, a lack of self-control and a significant negative reaction if the source is not obtained.

Addictions are treatable with a focus on breaking the cycle of motivation, cravings and reward. Depending on the source, specific self-help or mutual support groups are often recommended, particularly for illegal drugs and alcohol addictions. For a smoking addiction, nicotine replacement therapy (NRT) can be effective. During recovery, an individual might experience withdrawal symptoms, such as tremors, nausea, sweating or feeling anxious, so medication may be prescribed.

Addison's Disease

Addison's Disease is also called primary adrenal insufficiency or hypoadrenalism. It is a rare endocrine disorder that causes impairment to the adrenal glands, located atop the kidneys and responsible for the production of aldosterone and cortisol hormones. Extensive damage to the adrenal cortex, which surrounds the adrenal glands, causes the disease to develop, in the majority of cases as a result of an issue with the body's immune system. Other possible causes include infections, sepsis or cancer, and in less developed areas it has also been found that tuberculosis is responsible. Like other autoimmune diseases, genetic makeup can increase the risk of developing Addison's disease.

Symptoms are triggered when there is a lack of the correct level of cortisol and aldosterone. Habitually, they develop gradually over time and are akin to those of other conditions; tiredness and fatigue, reduced appetite leading to inadvertent weight loss, abdominal pain or weakness in the muscles. Dehydration and increased thirst are common, and as the disease develops, may be accompanied by vomiting, diarrhoea or fainting. Dark patches of skin (hyperpigmentation) may appear on the gums or where there are previous scars or natural creasing of the skin. Occasionally the onset of symptoms is rapid, signifying possible acute adrenal crisis which can be fatal if not treated immediately.

Corticosteroid replacement therapy to restore natural hormone levels is the primary treatment for Addison's disease – hydrocortisone is used for cortisol and fludrocortisone for aldosterone. Medication for this is typically taken a few times daily. Increasing salt in the diet can also potentially improve symptoms. It is advisable to wear a medical alert bracelet in case of an emergency adrenal crisis.

Allergies

Undeniably one of the most common conditions, allergies affect around a quarter of all people in the UK. The vast majority of allergies are considered mild, although they can still impact daily life. An allergy is caused when the body reacts to a particular substance, known as an allergen. They can develop at any point in a person's life. One of the most widespread allergies is hay fever, caused by grass and tree pollen. Within the medical environment, some allergies are triggered by certain types of medication (most commonly aspirin) or latex (found in some plasters or gloves).

The onset of allergy symptoms can happen in a few minutes' post-exposure to the allergen and are likely to worsen over a few hours; milder signs include sneezing, wheezing or coughing, a runny or blocked nose or itchy eyes. The skin may also be affected by a raised, itchy rash known as hives. In the case of food allergies, consumption of an allergen may result in stomach ache, nausea or vomiting. Anaphylaxis is the term used to describe a severe allergic reaction; when the body falls into anaphylactic shock it can be life threatening and medical intervention is required immediately. Symptoms can be almost instantaneous and include swelling, particularly of the throat and mouth which in turn can cause breathing difficulties, blue lips or skin (associated with a lack of blood circulation) or a loss of consciousness. Diagnosis can enable avoidance of a known allergen and depending on the cause, a range of specific medications are available to manage treatment, such as antihistamines, decongestants, lotions or steroids. For serious allergies, desensitisation to the allergen through immunotherapy may be explored as a more comprehensive treatment option.

Alzheimer's Disease

Alzheimer's Disease is a type of dementia, which impacts the functioning of the brain. The disease is caused by disrupted connections between nerve cells in the brain, impacted by a build-up of proteins (amyloid and tau) which result in abnormal structures known as plaques and tangles. These abnormalities cause a loss of brain tissue as the nerve cells die. There is also a reduction in certain chemical messengers (particularly low levels of acetylcholine) which are responsible for brain signals. Scientists are unclear why the process starts but as a progressive disease, the brain becomes more impacted and symptoms worsen over time. The biggest significant risk factor to having the disease is age; over 65 the chance of developing the condition doubles around every 5 years. Cases in women appear to be doubled when compared to men.

Often the first apparent symptom of Alzheimer's disease are memory lapses – losing items, forgetting names, dates, events or conversations. Secondary symptoms tend to impact speech, reasoning, concentration or perception but it can vary hugely depending on the individual. The later stages of Alzheimer's can be hugely distressing for those around them and whilst the individual may be particularly distressed, they may also be unaware of their behaviour. Symptoms can include hallucinations, delusions, difficulty with everyday tasks or acting out aggressively or in another manner that is not typical of them. An improvement in some symptoms can be seen with medication, specifically cholinesterase inhibitors, whilst tailored therapies and activities help with behavioural and psychological symptoms (BPSD).

Ankylosing Spondylitis

Ankylosing Spondylitis (AS) is a long-term condition that is almost twice as likely to be diagnosed in men than women. It affects the bones and joints of the lower spine, causing them to either fuse together or lose flexibility, resulting in pain for the individual. It is thought that the condition is genetic, found in families and passed down via the human leukocyte antigen B27 (HLA-B27) gene. The gene is not a predetermination of the disease, but it is carried in the vast majority of people with the condition.

The illness is different for everyone – symptoms tend to develop gradually and get worse over time, but they may also improve. Initial symptoms are typically seen in individuals between the ages of 20 and 30 and are commonly cited as pain and stiffness in the back and buttocks. Pain can be heightened in the morning and at night but may reduce with exercise and movement. The condition can cause symptoms of arthritis and enthesitis, inflammation of the joints, tendons or ligaments, as well as fatigue, leaving the individual lacking in energy. More severe cases can also lead to eye conditions, potential compression fractures or heart problems.

Unfortunately, there is no cure for the disease, but a combination of medication, physical therapy and exercise can help to control and potentially delay the stiffening of the spine and reduce the severity of the symptoms. Physical therapies such as massage techniques and hydrotherapy can complement daily stretching exercises, while anti-inflammatory medication can be approved to manage pain and reduce swelling.

Anxiety Disorders

Anxiety is a feeling of unease that most of us will experience at some point in our lives, triggered often by a situation that is unfamiliar or where there is perceived discomfort. However, when that feeling becomes constant and seemingly impossible to manage, it can be the main symptom of an anxiety disorder. There are six major types of anxiety disorders: separation anxiety disorder, specific phobias, social phobia, panic disorder, agoraphobia or generalised anxiety disorder (GAD). Unlike the others, GAD can be overwhelming to an individual as they experience worry or fear almost all of the time. Symptoms can be twofold, impacting both physical and mental health. Physical responses include insomnia, nausea or headaches, heart palpitations, muscles aches or a dry mouth. Psychological sensations can be felt as an unnerving sense of dread, lack of concentration and feeling constantly on edge. As the symptoms align to many other conditions, GAD can be hard to diagnose, especially as there is no obvious trigger or cause.

Usually, the first line of treatment for generalised anxiety disorder is a range of psychological interventions and therapies. Cognitive behavioural therapy (CBT) helps to directly question and explore the emotions and feelings around the individual's anxiety, whilst guided meditation and applied relaxation focus on relaxing muscles and preventing tension. Medication is also an option on both a short and longer-term basis. Antidepressants (SSRIs or SNRIs) or an anticonvulsant (pregabalin) are the most popular and generally used for milder symptoms; alternatively, a type of sedative called benzodiazepine can be diagnosed to treat severe symptoms in the immediate short-term.

Arachnoiditis

The arachnoid is one of the membranes surrounding the spinal cord – if it becomes inflamed it can cause arachnoiditis, a painful condition that is difficult to treat due to its inconsistent symptoms. There is no definitive cause of arachnoiditis, but the symptoms are often considered the result of previous trauma, injury or infections of the spinal cord. Approximately half of all cases are attributed to complications from previous spinal surgery. There have also been cases linked with the use of chemicals, such as those found in steroid injections.

There are no consistent signs of arachnoiditis which can make it hard to diagnose. The primary symptom is chronic pain, which can be experienced as a stinging or burning pain at a point in the lower back, not too dissimilar to an electric shock sensation. For some it might be muscle cramps or spasms; for others it may be tingling or numbness. Less common symptoms can include a distressing, itchy sensation not dissimilar to insects crawling under the skin. Activity can aggravate the pain and make it worse. There is no obvious cure for arachnoiditis, only treatment to manage and hopefully reduce the chronic pain. These include physical therapy and a pain management plan. Some claim that the pain felt by those with arachnoiditis is psychosomatic – solely in their head – and as such psychotherapy can be a tool for addressing symptoms of soreness. Surgery tends to be controversial due to the potential for further complications and enhanced scar tissue, both of which can be considered the cause of the disorder.

Arthritis

There are a number of types of arthritis; all affect the joints within the body and cause a level of pain. Whilst some types are more prevalent in older people, the disease can affect individuals of all ages. The probability of developing arthritis can be hereditary, so there is an increased risk if parents or grandparents have the condition.

Osteoarthritis is the most prevalent type. More likely to affect women and those beyond their mid-40s, it develops as a result of cartilage lining thinning out, causing swelling and extra segments of bone (osteophytes) to form. In turn this results in stiffness and pain. Rheumatoid arthritis tends to emerge between the ages of 40 and 50, also affecting more women, and is an auto-immune condition; the body's immune system attacks the joints, leading to a breakdown of cartilage. Other well-known types of arthritis include ankylosing spondylitis, fibromyalgia, lupus and gout. With several types come numerous symptoms but regular to most is pain, weakness or tenderness in the joints, visible inflammation or difficulty moving the affected area.

Treatment for arthritis is largely about managing the pain and keeping the joints as strong as possible. Low-impact exercise, such as swimming, cycling or yoga, combined with physiotherapy will help to build and maintain good muscle condition and keep joints moving within the correct range. Maintaining a healthy body weight will ensure there is less unnecessary impact on the joints. Medication called DMARDs or biological medicines can be diagnosed to limit the effects of rheumatoid arthritis. For serious damage from osteoarthritis, surgery to repair or replace an impaired joint might be feasible.

Asperger's Syndrome

Asperger's Syndrome is technically the same diagnosis as that of autism spectrum disorder (ASD), although it is typically less severe. As autism is a spectrum condition, rather than a disease or illness, individuals who have been given a diagnosis will be affected in different ways; they will experience the world around them differently to the majority of people. More often than not the first symptoms will become noticeable during childhood, particularly with the development of social skills; a child may not pick up on social cues (body language, facial expressions or tone of voice) like their peers or appear to display very few emotions. Repetitive comments or movements are common and so is the intense interest in a particular subject, often intellectual or artistic.

There are no cures or specific treatments for Asperger's syndrome or ASD. Depending on an individual's symptoms they may require varying degrees of support. Working with the symptoms, rather than against them, can help to ease them; for example, setting routines and sticking to them to reduce change and unpredictability, or reducing the amount of social expectation by allocating alone time. Guidance from medical professionals may recommend treatments such as social skills training or applied behaviour analysis to nurture positive communication techniques. Medication is only available to help treat related symptoms such as anxiety, depression or ADHD.

Asthma

Asthma is a common condition which depending on the severity can either be a minor irritant or a major, potentially life-threatening issue. In children it affects more boys than girls but that is reversed in adults, with more women being diagnosed. It is understood that genetics play a factor in the cause, along with modern-day pollution and sanitation levels.

Asthma is a physical reaction to a personal trigger, either external, such as pollution, cigarette smoke, mould and damp, pets, dust mites and pollen, or internal, due to emotions, stress, anxiety or chest infections. It is possible to have multiple triggers.

Airways carrying air to and from the lungs are surrounded by muscles, which tighten and can cause the tubes to become narrow. Swelling and inflammation can occur, whilst a build-up of phlegm can further reduce the size of the airway. This leads to the onset of asthma symptoms, including wheezing, coughing and breathlessness. If the symptoms develop it can cause an asthma attack leading to breathing difficulties. At this point immediate medical intervention is typically required. Other external factors such as hormonal changes or being pregnant, both of which can aggravate or improve the asthmatic symptoms.

It is managed through the use of inhalers, a contraption to enable the inhalation of medication. There are 3 types of inhaler – reliever inhalers (to relieve symptoms within a few minutes as and when they arise) which are usually blue in colour, preventer inhalers (taken daily to help prevent the impact of triggers) and combination inhalers which contain both. For more acute cases, further treatment can be provided through medication, injections administered every few weeks, or even bronchial thermoplasty surgery.

Attention Deficit Hyperactivity Disorder (ADHD)

Commonly known by its acronym ADHD, Attention Deficit Hyperactivity Disorder is typically associated with children and most diagnoses are made when a child is between 6 and 12 years of age. It is a neurodevelopmental behavioural disorder which appears to run in families and therefore genetics are believed to increase the risk of developing the condition. There is also some scientific evidence that brain structure and the chemicals within it may contribute to causing ADHD.

Symptoms seen in children fall into two categories: inattentiveness, and hyperactivity and impulsiveness. Behaviours indicative of inattentiveness include distraction and a lack of focus, interrupting others, being forgetful or unable to concentrate or listen to instructions. The key indicators of hyperactivity and impulsiveness are constant fidgeting or the inability to sit still, poor concentration, excessive talking or moving and acting before thinking (and therefore having little sense of potential danger). If an individual only presents symptoms of inattentiveness without hyperactivity and impulsiveness, attention deficit disorder (ADD) will be diagnosed instead. Symptoms can persist through to adulthood, though may impact the individual in a slightly more complex manner; for example, an inability to deal with stress, mood swings, restlessness, lack of attention to detail or a short attention span or extreme impatience.

A combination of medication and therapy is often best in treating the symptoms. There are 5 types of medication, the more common ones are stimulants that can be taken either daily or just on school days (depending on the severity of the condition). Behaviour therapy, social skills training or psychoeducation can be partnered with parent training to offer a well-rounded support programme.

Autism

As a spectrum condition, Autism symptoms can vary both in range and severity and as such diagnosis can be extremely broad – some people need little assistance whereas others might require constant support. There is no clear cause of autism, but it is believed that both physical factors coupled with genetics are key, as multiple diagnoses can be found within the same family. It is also three times as likely to be seen in men than women. Those with autism might also be diagnosed with other conditions, such as epilepsy, ADHD or a mental health disorder. Problems with social communication and social interaction are the two key signals of autism. Challenges with understanding and interpreting certain verbal and non-verbal cues can lead to the belief that autistic people are insensitive or socially inappropriate. Some individuals have limited speech and language or find it hard to process concepts such as jokes and sarcasm as they find it hard to read other people's feelings and intentions. Social interaction can be overwhelming and require time spent alone. Some physical symptoms include an increased or decreased sensitivity in their response to pain, temperatures, sounds, smells, touches or tastes. Repetitive behaviour patterns known as stimming, such as clicking a pen or rocking in a chair, can reduce stress or extreme anxiety. Other characteristics are a seeming fixation on particular interests or hobbies and a meltdown or shutdown in response to becoming completely overwhelmed. There are numerous fake treatments that claim to help 'cure' people from autism; in reality there is no cure, but there are a number of biomedical interventions and therapy options available to help manage the individual symptoms and support an autistic person to thrive.

Benign Prostatic Hyperplasia

A condition found only in men, Benign Prostatic Hyperplasia (BPH) is a swelling of the prostate gland. Also known as prostate enlargement, it is a relatively common condition diagnosed over the age of 50 and seen as a normal ageing process in men over the age of 80. As hormones change over a person's lifetime, it is this natural process that may be a factor in the cause of prostate enlargement. Due to the added pressure an enlarged prostate has on the bladder and urethra, common symptoms have an impact on urination, such as the frequent need to pee or difficulty in starting or finishing. Nocturia (needing to urinate multiple times during the night), painful urination or spotting blood in the urine are also signs that there might be something wrong. If left untreated, symptoms can become more serious and develop into further issues such as kidney failure, persistent urinary tract infections or incontinence.

Regular medical check-ups are advisable to keep the symptoms under control and minimise the risk of them getting worse. Lifestyle changes, such as a reduction in alcohol, regular exercise and limiting the consumption of artificial sweeteners, can have a positive impact on symptoms. Other self-care methods can include a concerted effort to reduce stress levels or practicing Kegel exercises, specifically targeting and strengthening pelvic muscles. Medication can be used to treat moderate to severe cases and where no impact is seen, surgery can be considered to directly address more serious symptoms such as incontinence, kidney failure or recurrent urinary tract infections.

Bipolar Disorder

Bipolar disorder is a chronic mental health condition that usually commences during teenage years or early adulthood. As well as being five times more likely to develop the condition if a family member has it, another probable cause is chemical imbalances within the brain. Environmental and social triggers, for instance a relationship breakdown, any form of abuse, grief or a physical illness, can lead to the symptoms of bipolar disorder.

Once referred to as manic depression, bipolar disorder has two main categories of symptoms: mania and depression. Unlike most people who experience general ups and downs in their emotions, those with bipolar feel them intensely and swing between the extremes. Characteristics synonymous with mania are feelings of elated happiness, an emphasis on self-importance, making big, rash decisions or being seemingly full of grand, exciting ideas. On the flip side, symptoms of a depressive episode include feelings of hopelessness, emptiness or sadness, guilt or despair, and physical indicators such as a loss of appetite or energy and difficulty sleeping. Episodes can last for weeks or months and there are different categories of the disorder, depending on the frequency and the severity of the symptoms. Some might also encounter hallucinogenic or delusional psychotic symptoms. Treatment is generally quite encouraging though may take some trial and error to establish the best method for the individual. Mood stabilising medication can be taken regularly (the most common is lithium), enhanced with relevant medication during a manic or depressive episode. Psychological treatments can also help to notice patterns and triggers that may enable better management of the episodes prior to or at the onset.

Body Dysmorphic Disorder

Classified as an anxiety disorder, Body Dysmorphic Disorder (BDD) is embodied by distorted thoughts and excessive concern about one's own physical appearance. Sometimes referred to as body dysmorphia, BDD affects both men and women, primarily older children and young adults. A myriad of factors can increase the risk of developing the disorder, including bullying, societal or peer pressure, perfectionism, genetics or other mood disorders.

As those diagnosed with BDD see themselves in a different way to how others are likely to, symptoms of the disorder include undue worries about self-image and frequent comparison with other people's looks. Physically it can cause an individual to develop obsessive, compulsive behaviours, such as excessive use of mirrors, regular styling or use of intense make-up, or picking at skin in an attempt to try and improve its appearance. There can be similarities drawn between BDD and eating disorders, though BDD tends to be associated with a general body image or specific body area, rather than weight and body shape.

The first line of treatment is typically talking therapies, specifically cognitive behavioural therapy (CBT) to help identify the potential thoughts and behaviours around the disorder. A particular technique known as exposure and response prevention (ERP) might be suggested, exposing the individual to the situation where they are likely to display symptoms and developing coping strategies to overcome them. Antidepressant medications, most likely a serotonin-specific reuptake inhibitor (SSRI) or clomipramine, may also be prescribed to minimise compulsive thoughts and actions.

Borderline Personality Disorder

One of a group of wider personality disorders, Borderline Personality Disorder (BPD) is related to emotions, thought processes, behaviour and interpersonal interactions. Of those diagnosed, approximately three quarters are women, though it is not apparent why this is the case. The causes of BPD are cited as a combination of genetic factors, impacted brain development or altered levels of brain chemicals, and traumatic childhood experiences, such as neglect, abuse, grief or instability within the family.

Symptoms are largely categorised into four areas. It is sometimes named emotionally unstable personality disorder (EUPD) and volatile emotions are characteristic of BPD, with intense mood swings not being uncommon. It may include feelings of despair or loneliness, leading to suicidal thoughts, switching to more positive emotions in a cyclical nature (known as affective dysregulation). Thinking or cognitive patterns can also be distorted, leading to disturbing beliefs that result in seemingly risky behaviour such as self-harm or using alcohol or drugs to numb the emotions. A fear of abandonment is central to BPD, which can result in trust issues, unstable relationships and 'black-and-white thinking' (splitting) that people are either all good or all bad. Therapy is the most widely regarded form of treatment for BPD, particularly dialectal behaviour therapy (DBT) which is specifically designed to acknowledge emotional vulnerability, validate negative emotions and break the cycle of detrimental behaviour. Mentalisation-based therapy (MBT) will consider an individual's mental state, and that of those around them, whilst arts therapies help to express emotions without the medium of talking.

Brittle Bone Disease

Brittle Bone Disease, or osteogenesis imperfecta ("imperfectly formed bone"), is a genetic disorder that affects all bones in the human body and is usually diagnosed during early childhood. The presence of a protein called type 1 collagen enables bones to grow and develop; brittle bone disease is caused by a defect, mutation or change in one of the four genes that is responsible for collagen production. There is no bias towards either men or women and it is found equally among all ethnic groups.

As expected from its name, the main symptom of the disease is weak, brittle bones that break very easily. Due to their fragility, there can also be deformities within the bones leading to weak and loose joints, bowed arms and legs or an abnormal curvature of the spine. Further symptoms can impact the respiratory system, hearing, muscles and tissues whilst also leading to easily damaged skin, bleeding and bruising.

Whilst there is no known cure for brittle bone disease, a range of treatments can improve quality of life and reduce the impact of the disease. Medication can be administered to both strengthen bones and reduce potential pain, whilst physical therapy helps to improve the condition and can be complemented by casts, braces and splints for weak or broken bones. For serious cases, surgery is an option – either inserting rods to support the bones or reconstruction of bone deformities. Maintaining a healthy, balanced diet, doing regular low-impact exercise and avoiding alcohol and smoking can also help to improve symptoms.

Bronchiectasis

Relatively uncommon and with symptoms typically developing in middle age and beyond, Bronchiectasis is a long-term lung condition usually caused by previous damage to tissue and muscles in the airways. Lungs become inflamed with a build-up of phlegm and mucus in the bronchi (and smaller bronchioles) and without the usual bodily defence mechanisms to keep them clear, it can easily develop into an infection. There is not always an evident underlying cause, but it has been linked to the development from previous lung infections such as pneumonia, tuberculosis or whooping cough. Bronchiectasis is also sometimes known as non-cystic fibrosis bronchiectasis. The most common symptoms include breathlessness and a constant, relentless cough which brings up sputum or phlegm – both of which can be a sign of a more serious lung condition. Other less common symptoms include sinus problems, feeling lethargic, coughing up blood or chest pain. A diagnosis is typically made after a series of tests including a chest X-ray, CT scan and lung function tests.

A range of treatments are utilised to limit further development of the illness, as well as treat and help relieve the symptoms. A respiratory physiotherapist may administer breathing exercise to assist with airway clearance. Some people are prone to frequent chest infections and may require regular courses of antibiotics to keep them from flaring up. Surgery is extremely uncommon in the treatment of the condition but can be considered in cases where usual therapies have proved to be unsuccessful.

Cancer

With over 200 different cancer varieties, the condition is growing increasingly more widespread; recent studies suggest that approximately half of the population will develop one form of cancer or another during their life cycle. There are multiple possible causes; a genetic predisposition of gene mutations, combined biological and lifestyle factors is thought to be the most likely. Exposure to harmful chemicals or radiation can also be a trigger. Living a healthy lifestyle can substantially lessen an individual's chance of developing cancer, particularly having a nutritious, balanced diet and avoiding habits such as smoking and drinking alcohol excessively.

The condition can be very slow to progressively develop so remain unseen with no visible symptoms for many years. It starts due to the presence of abnormal cells that reproduce and divide in an uncontrolled manner. In time this can result in a lump or growth known as a tumour, which is often the primary indication that cancer may be present. In addition, there may be noticeable changes in typical bowel patterns, unexplainable bleeding or frequent bloating or the appearance of moles on the skin. Dependent on the type of cells involved, cancers can be categorised into various different types: carcinomas (skin or tissue), sarcomas (bone or muscle), lymphomas (vessels or glands), leukaemias (cancers of the blood) or brain tumours. Some have the ability to spread further throughout the body. With the correct treatment, cancers can be slowed, stopped and often cured. A solid tumour may be removed via a surgical procedure. Chemotherapy, a form of cancer medication, or radiotherapy, the use of X-rays to destroy the cancerous cells, are both forms of sessional treatment that aim to destroy the cancerous cells.

Charcot-Marie-Tooth Disease

Sometimes referred to as peroneal muscular atrophy, or hereditary motor and sensory neuropathy, Charcot-Marie-Tooth disease (CMT) is a condition that causes damage to the nerves that control senses and movement. It is a group of disorders caused by genetic mutations inherited from either one or both parents; depending on the type of mutation, one of five different types of CMT can be caused. The specific nerves that are affected are peripheral nerves, which link the brain to the central nervous system.

Symptoms are highly varied but likely to first appear during adolescence and often start with weakness or numbness in the lower limbs, including legs, ankles and feet. Often the individual will have symptoms that affect their gait, such as footdrop, unusually high arches, flat feet or hammer toes. The arms and hands can also be impacted, chiefly as a result of weakness and poor circulation. As CMT is a progressive condition, the symptoms can worsen over time, particularly posture and mobility problems, dexterity and muscle strength.

Whilst there is no known cure for CMT, due to the speed at which the disease progress, treatment is aimed at managing the symptoms on a daily basis. Regular assessments conducted by a multidisciplinary team ensure that symptoms are monitored and given the best possible treatment. Physiotherapy techniques, including limb manipulation and massage, is often combined with occupational therapy which can address the use of adaptive aid to improve quality of life. To aid gait and mobility, orthopaedic devices such as splints, braces or orthotic innersoles may be used. Surgery may be used to correct major deformities.

Chronic Fatigue Syndrome

Chronic Fatigue Syndrome (CFS) is also known as myalgic encephalomyelitis (ME) so is often referred to as CFS/ME. It impacts more women than men and the specific cause remains unknown – though concepts of viral or bacterial infections, immune system complications, hormonal imbalances and mental health problems have been suggested as potential triggers.

The main trait is an extreme fatigue that frustratingly for the individual, no amount of rest or sleep will improve. The onset of exhaustion tends to show between mid-20s and mid-40s. Additional symptoms can include muscular and joint pain or flu-like symptoms, restless sleep, nausea, concentration or memory problems and occasionally heart palpitations. CFS/ME can easily impact daily activities and even minimal physical or mental exertion may bring about post-exertional malaise (PEM), a worsening of the general symptoms. In major cases it can leave individuals completely bedbound. Symptoms can improve by themselves over time and for many people, this is the case, but for others there are a range of therapies available to help relieve the seriousness. Graded exercise therapy (GET) assists in gradually increasing physical activity to a level that is achievable to the individual. Cognitive behavioural therapy can address the underlying thought processes surrounding the condition and help to reframe its presence in the person's life. Some appropriate lifestyle changes may also be recommended to improve and reduce certain symptoms, for example, maintaining a healthy, balanced diet, adopting routines and taking over-the-counter medicines to relieve common symptoms such as headaches and muscular pain.

Chronic Obstructive Pulmonary Disease

Often referred to as COPD, Chronic Obstructive Pulmonary Disease is a group of inflammatory conditions, the main two being emphysema and chronic bronchitis, that directly affect the lungs. The former refers to damage of the air sacs (alveoli) within the lungs and the latter occurs as a result of inflammation of the tubes (bronchioles).

The most significant cause that is attributable to around 90% of cases is smoking – toxic chemicals cause damage to the lungs, even from exposure to second-hand smoke. Dust and fumes from chemicals, food or other substances, as well as increased pollution in the air, can cause irritation and lead to the onset of COPD symptoms. There is also a far greater chance of developing the condition if there is a deficiency in the gene alpha-1-antitypsin.

Symptoms generally emerge after substantial damage has already been caused to the lungs. One of the most obvious is a lingering, chesty cough, partnered with wheezing, shortness of breath or a tight chest. A less obvious indication is unexplained weight loss or swelling of the ankles due to an accumulation of fluid (known as oedema). If smoking or exposure to smoke persists, then symptoms are likely to continue to get worse.

Stopping smoking is the primary method of improving the condition, using addiction support if required, and a specialist exercise programme called pulmonary rehabilitation can assist with the breathlessness. Appropriate medication can be administered in the form of tablets or inhalers to help deal with flare ups and in a minute number of cases, a lung transplant may be required.

Chronic Pain Syndrome

Everyone will experience pain at some point; it is the body's natural response to illness or injury. After the healing process the pain usually ceases but for many people it can persist for much longer – when it is still present 3-6 months later it is classified as chronic pain. In turn this can cause further complications and it then develops into a condition called Chronic Pain Syndrome. Some other health conditions are highly likely to be cited as a cause of chronic pain; fibromyalgia, arthritis, inflammatory bowel disease or trauma sustained as a result of surgery.

Physical symptoms of the condition can manifest as muscular or joint aches and pains (sometimes dull, sometimes burning or intense), fatigue and a loss of strength. It is likely to also impact mentally and emotionally, from sleep disorders and mood swings to mental health problems such as depression. The chronic pain cycle can be devastating to the individual – the pain itself can bring on other issues and in turn make it even harder to deal with the pain. Occasionally there can sometimes be no known trigger for the pain, instead simply a miscommunication between the nervous system and the brain. Where there is a known cause, treatment is carried out by a specialist in that area. If the pain is present in a specific area, physical therapy such as massage or transcutaneous electrical nerve stimulation (TENS) can help to reduce it. Occupational therapy or counselling can enable someone to manage the complications of living with pain on a daily basis. A whole range of medication may also be suitable, although there is a risk of addiction depending on the frequency with which it is relied upon.

Chronic Exertional Compartment Syndrome

Compartment syndrome is a painful condition caused by an increased pressure within the compartment, a contained bundle of muscles, blood vessels and nerves. Unlike Acute Compartment Syndrome, which is usually caused by a severe injury and considered a medical emergency, Chronic Exertional Compartment Syndrome (CECS) happens more gradually with the onset of exercise. The cause of CECS is unknown and it can be notoriously difficult to diagnose. During exercise, muscles will swell and may impact the blood supply, bringing on the symptoms. A range of physical examinations may be used to obtain a diagnosis, including post-exercise imaging scans or compartment pressure measurements.

The main symptom is a cramp or pain brought on soon after starting a repetitive exercise such as walking, running or cycling. The muscle may visibly bulge, and most people will experience tenderness, tingling or a constant, nagging pain which usually desists when exercise is stopped. The legs are most commonly affected but it can also be found in the arms, hands or feet.

A reduction in or complete end to the exercise that initiates pain is often the only way to reduce symptoms. Physiotherapy, gait analysis and orthotic aids may assist, whilst anti-inflammatory medication can be taken to reduce the pain when it occurs. Surgery can be considered in cases where other non-invasive treatments have proved unsuccessful. A procedure called a fasciotomy is conducted to open the fascia (the tissue surrounding the muscle compartments) and relieve pressure.

Coeliac Disease

Gluten is a family of proteins found in wheat, barley, and rye cereals, commonly found in the everyday food that we consume including pasta, bread, cakes and biscuits, breakfast cereals and alcohol. For someone with Coeliac Disease, when gluten is consumed, their body's immune system will attack its own tissues. Not considered an intolerance or food allergy, coeliac disease is a serious autoimmune condition that can cause damage to the gut and have significant consequences on the body's ability to absorb nutrients. It is relatively common, with 1 in 100 people affected. If a direct family member has the disease the odds increase to 1 in 10. It tends to affect around two thirds more women than men and symptoms have a tendency to develop in early childhood or later adulthood, after the age of 40.

There are a range of symptoms displayed in the gut, including stomach aches, diarrhoea, indigestion and constipation. A long-term lack of nutrients can lead to complications such as vitamin B12 and folate and iron deficiency anaemia.

The best way to manage coeliac disease is to adopt a balanced, healthy gluten-free diet. Within a few weeks of cutting out gluten, symptoms should ease and the digestive system can start to heal. An increasing variety of gluten-free foods are being manufactured to assist with daily management of the condition. Vitamin and mineral supplements may be prescribed by a medical professional to ensure the body receives the vital nutrients it needs.

Complex Regional Pain Syndrome

Complex Regional Pain Syndrome (CRPS) has two subtypes: reflex sympathetic dystrophy (type 1) and causalgia (type 2). The syndrome is embodied by a chronic, disproportionate level of pain, either stemming from a specific injury or illness or, in the case of causalgia, from damage to the nerves. It is not abundantly clear why this happens, though the most cited suggestion is that various body systems — such as the central nervous system or the immune system — have an abnormal, malfunctional response. Inflammation may also bring about the syndrome and there is evidence that psychological factors can also exacerbate the symptoms. It is less common in children and tends to affect women more than men. Pain is usually felt at the sight of the pre-existing injury but can stretch to the rest of the limb or even beyond. Typically, it commences within a month or so post-injury and encompasses swelling and tenderness with an intense, burning pain that can feel akin to stabbing. It can be caused by a seemingly insignificant touch or bump (hyperalgesia) or a gentle stroke along the skin (allodynia). This is the acute phase which usually lasts for a few months, followed by the dystrophic phase when there are visible changes to the skin, stiffening and turning shiny. If it develops into the atrophic stage, then function and motion of the limb might be compromised due to muscle wastage.

Most individuals will see an improvement in symptoms within 2 years' post-injury. Rehabilitation of the area utilises techniques such as desensitisation, graded motor imagery and mirror visual feedback to help reorient the brain. A range of medication can be used and a focus on psychological support and wellbeing is important for long-term pain management.

Crohn's Disease

Along with ulcerative colitis, Crohn's Disease is one of the two forms of Inflammatory Bowel Disease (IBD). It affects the digestive system, or gut, causing swelling which impacts the body's ability to digest food and absorb nutrients. The chance of having the disease is part in due to genetics and part in due to other internal factors including an issue with the immune system or an imbalance of gut bacteria. It is believed that smoking also increases the chances. The indicative symptoms are generally first seen during childhood or early adulthood. Signs that the condition may be present include stomach cramps, diarrhoea (sometimes mixed with pus or blood), fatigue and loss of appetite leading to a loss of weight. Other indicators might be regular mouth ulcers, feeling sick and patchy areas of a rash, usually found on the legs. Some people might experience their symptoms constantly whereas for others they may disappear and return every few weeks or months (a cycle of relapses and remission).

In terms of treatment, medication is the primary method of targeting the symptoms. Steroids, taken as tablets or sometimes injections, can lessen the inflammation in the gut, and immunosuppressant medicines can help to reduce negative activity from the body's immune system. Some individuals may be prescribed a liquid diet (enteral nutrition) for several weeks – it contains all the required nutrients but will allow time for the symptoms to hopefully lessen. In other cases, a surgical procedure called a resection can be conducted, removing damaged sections of the bowel, and joining the surrounding healthy parts together. However, results from surgery may only be temporary.

Cystic Fibrosis

Cystic Fibrosis is a purely inherited condition and therefore indicators can be present even before birth (picked up using antenatal testing) but usually at the point of birth (tested for using the standard heel-prick test). Around 1 in 25 of adults in the UK carry the faulty gene, often unknown to themselves. A genetic test and sweat test – to determine if there is an unusually high level of salt – are the standard methods to confirm a diagnosis.

Cystic fibrosis initiates a thick, sticky mucus to be produced within the body which targets the lungs and sometimes the pancreas, responsible for food digestion. Because of this, breathing is hindered and causes coughing, wheezing, chest infections and potential destruction of the airways (bronchiectasis). If the pancreas becomes clogged it can result in issues with normal absorption of nutrients from food and lead to malnutrition and troubles with growing and reaching a normal body weight. Other symptoms also include jaundice or bowel problems such as diarrhoea or constipation.

A range of treatments are available to manage the everyday symptoms but there is no cure for cystic fibrosis. Medication targets infections in the chest and helps to thin or reduce the level of mucus causing the damage. It is also advisable to have the flu vaccination each year. A physiotherapist will advise on airway clearance techniques as well as other forms of physical activity which help to clear the mucus, whilst a dietician will assist if malnutrition becomes apparent. If damage to the lungs has resulted in them not working properly then surgery for a lung transplant may be considered – this is usually only in profoundly serious cases as it carries a number of risks.

Depression

Depression is often a misunderstood condition due to the perceived familiarity of the symptoms – low moods and feeling sad or fed up. Almost everyone has experienced those emotions at some point, but depression can leave an individual feeling them intensely for a prolonged period. There are numerous, varied causes of depression and reasons for being at a higher risk of developing it – stressful events (such as bereavement, job losses, relationship issues or money troubles), family history, social isolation and loneliness, pregnancy and giving birth (postnatal depression), illness or injury or even specific personality types.

Low mood is the main symptom but usually partnered with feelings of worthlessness or guilt, a loss of self-esteem, numbness and emptiness, losing interest in hobbies and feeling lethargic and tired. It can result in social avoidance, sleep disorders or eating disorders and physical aches and pains. Some people may experience psychotic symptoms such as paranoia and hallucinations and at its worst, depression can lead to thoughts of self-harm and suicide.

It is recommended that medical support is sought after symptoms have been experienced incessantly for over at least 2 continuous weeks. In the first instance self-help might be recommended – doing daily exercise, using talking therapies online or seeking out local support groups – and there are a number of talking therapies including CBT, counselling, interpersonal therapy or psychodynamic psychotherapy. Whilst there is currently no solid evidence that a chemical imbalance in the brain causes depression, antidepressant medication helps balance chemicals and can reduce some of the symptoms.

Dermatomyositis

Dermatomyositis (DM) is a form of myositis, a group of rare conditions that are symptomatic of muscle weakness and pain. It is around twice as common in women than in men and whilst it can affect any age group, juvenile dermatomyositis is a more specific form when found in children. There is no clear cause of dermatomyositis but like the other forms, indicators suggest it is as a result of both environmental and genetic factors. There is some thought that it could be the result of a viral infection but the most renowned concept is that it is an autoimmune disease, whereby the body's natural defence system mistakenly attacks its own cells and tissues.

As the name 'derma' (meaning 'skin') suggests, the main distinguishing symptom of dermatomyositis is a dark red or violet coloured patchy irritation on the skin called a heliotrope rash. It usually appears first on the face, around the eyelids, or around the knuckles on the hands, caused by swollen blood vessels. As with other types of myositis, muscles are also tender and weak, often starting with the larger ones found in the shoulders and hips. Movement can be difficult and painful, and the throat can also be impacted making it difficult to swallow or altering the voice.

Steroids and immunosuppressant medication are used to treat the inflammation and reduce the immune system's chances of muscle damage. In rare situations immunoglobulin therapy may be considered, providing the body with an injection of healthy antibodies from donated plasma. The condition can impact daily activities but regular, strengthening exercise is important to keep the muscles growing strong and healthy.

Diabetes

Diabetes causes the glucose level in the blood to become too high. There are a number of different variations of diabetes; most people are diagnosed with either type 1 or type 2.

A hormone called insulin, made by the pancreas, is responsible for fuelling the body by allowing glucose to enter the cells. When the pancreas is unable to produce any insulin at all, this is indicative of type 1 diabetes. Type 2 diabetes is more common, accountable for around 90% of all diabetes diagnoses in the UK. It happens when the pancreas is unable to produce enough insulin (or what it does produce is not effective). The chances of developing it increase for an individual if a close relative has the condition, is from an Asia, African-Caribbean or black African origin, is over the age of 40 or is overweight or obese. A condition called prediabetes is a good indicator of an increased risk of developing type 2 diabetes.

Symptoms are similar but those of type 1 diabetes can appear suddenly as opposed to over a number of months or years. They include extreme thirst and needing to urinate more than usual (especially at night), recurring thrush, blurred vision, unexplained weight loss and cuts or abrasions that take a long time to heal.

Type 1 diabetics need to take injections of insulin on a daily basis to keep the blood sugar levels under control. Type 2 diabetes is treated using a medication to lower blood sugar levels. There is also strong evidence that keeping fit and active is essential to keep the glucose levels down and an annual medical check-up is vital to ensure there are no further complications with cholesterol or blood pressure.

Dissociation and Dissociative Disorders

Feeling disconnected or detached, either from the outside world or from yourself, is known as Dissociation. It is a natural coping reaction from the mind, usually in response to significant trauma or stress, and can be a temporary state. However, when it is ongoing or to the point that it impacts an individual's daily life, it could be indication of a Dissociative Disorder. These disorders can develop when there are multiple periods of dissociation triggered from either ongoing or specific trauma, neglect or abuse, often experienced in childhood. Unlike a typical defence mechanism of fight or flight, it is also possible to 'freeze' (causing the body to go numb or unable to move) or 'flop' (thought processes are closed down and muscles become limp).

There are a few different dissociative disorders. Dissociative identity disorder (DID), previously known as multiple personality disorder, is characterised by uncertainty or memory loss about personal identity or the presence of multiple identities. Indicators of derealisation and depersonalisation disorder are a sensation of being on the outside, looking inwards on the self. For some people, the world may be foggy or not appear real. The main symptoms of dissociative amnesia are forgetfulness around personal identity or life events. It is possible to also experience a fugue, a complete loss of memory about the self which can lead to the temporary adoption of a new identity.

People may have multiple dissociative disorders at one time and with the relevant treatment, may be able to reduce the symptoms so that they are in control of their sense of self. Treatment is typically a combination of medication (antidepressants or antipsychotic medication), EMDR and talking therapies.

Dyslexia

Approximately 1 in 10 people in the UK has a level of Dyslexia, a learning disorder that impacts reading, writing, language and speech. It has no effect on intelligence, unlike most other learning disabilities. As a condition often found in families, the cause of dyslexia is believed to be linked to certain genes as well as environmental factors such as exposure to risks during pregnancy or premature birth.

Initial indicators of dyslexia may be apparent in young, pre-school children – problems with speech, slow development of talking or finding it difficult to form words correctly (for example, confusion between similar words or reversing sounds). By the time a child starts school, symptoms are likely to come more apparent in comparison to peers; they may be reading, spelling or writing at a lower level than expected for their age or they may be presenting memory problems. Sometimes a child with dyslexia will try to avoid reading or writing activities altogether. Dyslexia has a close association with ADHD, with children at increased risk of having both conditions. Similar issues can follow into teenage years and adulthood, developing into problems such as mispronunciation or misspelling of words, difficulty in summarising or memorising information, and trouble with working out mathematical problems.

Dyslexia can stunt learning and cause long-term educational and socio-economic issues. Support is managed through a range of dedicated educational interventions – most can be provided during mainstream education, but specialist schools exist for children with more acute difficulties. A focus is placed on phonological skills to help improve the processing of words and sounds, often aided by technology.

Dyspraxia

Sometimes confused with dyslexia, Dyspraxia is a condition that causes problems with physical motor coordination skills. Also known as developmental coordination disorder (DCD), dyspraxia is believed to affect boys around 3 to 4 times more than girls and be at higher risk if born prematurely. A disruption in the messaging between brain and body is believed to be the main cause. The first noticeable symptoms are generally a lag in reaching normal developmental milestones such as certain types of play, using cutlery to eat or learning to walk. As children get older, they may have issues with motor skills and coordination, impacting their ability to take part in usual playground activities or keeping still when required. Tasks requiring fine motor skills, such as using a pencil, cutting with scissors or doing up shoelaces, can also present problems. These issues can follow through into adulthood, impacting the ability to play certain sports or learn skills such as driving or DIY. Other issues can impede further education or employment, such as trouble with concentration, planning and organising.

Whilst sometimes the symptoms reduce over time, the condition is usually present for the duration of life. For children, a paediatric occupational therapist can help develop skills for daily life, whilst an educational psychologist will focus on progressing learning; task-oriented or process-oriented approaches, or a combination of both, are found to be the most effective. Other specialist healthcare professionals may be consulted if there is a specific issue, for example, a speech and language therapist can recommend mouth exercises for improving the formation of sounds and words. If symptoms are still displayed as an adult, occupational therapy can help to make suitable adaptions.

Dystonia

Dystonia directly impacts the muscles within the body, causing them to contract uncontrollably and resulting in involuntarily spasms or repetitive movements. The area of the brain responsible for the coordination of movement, the basal ganglia, is thought to be linked with dystonia – damage to this area through an injury or infection could be the cause of the condition. Complications linked with trauma, stroke, cerebral palsy, multiple sclerosis or Parkinson's disease have also been cited.

Symptoms can be seen in one muscle (focal), a group of muscles (multifocal) or across the whole body (generalised). If it affects adjacent body parts, it is known as segmental dystonia and hemidystonia affects limbs on the same side of the body. Muscle spasms can be mild or extreme, resulting in twisted contortions or whole-body tremors. They may be painful and exasperated by stress. Sometimes the symptoms can be seen as uncontrolled blinking of the eyes (blepharospasm).

As a habitually lifelong condition, treatments for dystonia are regularly monitored. Where a specific muscle can be identified, botulinum toxin (known as Botox) is directly injected approximately every 3 months in order to impede the chemical that produce muscular contractions. Deep brain stimulation is a surgical route that entails the insertion of a small electrode into the brain which is linked to a stimulator inserted under the skin of the chest. Electrical signals travel to the brain and reduce convulsions in the muscles. Occasionally the individual might be able to control their own contraction using sensory trick – touch manoeuvres in different areas of the body that can help improve spasms where there may have been a known trigger.

Eating Disorders

Classified as both mental and physical conditions, Eating Disorders can impact an individual of any age, gender or background, though are most commonly diagnosed in young or teenage girls. They are likely to be caused by a complex combination of genetic, environmental, sociocultural and psychological factors, such as family history, peer or societal pressure and perceived stigma around weight or dissatisfaction with body image.

There are a number of types of eating disorder. Anorexia nervosa is characterised by significant low weight, caused by a restriction of food, as well as weight loss, issues maintaining a healthy weight and often distorted body image. Binge eating disorder is related to uncontrollable bouts of eating, with associated shame or guilt about large portions or unhealthy habits. Similarly, an individual with bulimia nervosa is likely to be in a cycle of binge eating and then purging – purposefully inducing sickness or bowel movements (by taking laxative medicines), disproportionately exercising or fasting to offset the binge. Other specified feeding or eating disorder (OSFED), where symptoms are not completely aligned with the criteria to be diagnosed with anorexia, bulimia or binge eating, is the most common eating disorder. Avoidant/restrictive food intake disorder (ARFID) is generally associated with a specific or type of food.

Early intervention is key in the treatment of all eating disorders, particularly anorexia which can be life-threatening. Different types of tailored talking therapy are usually considered for the individual, and sometimes for those close to them too. Depending on the disorder, guided help or group support can be powerful in promoting recovery.

Ehlers-Danlos Syndrome

Ehlers-Danlos Syndrome (EDS) can be classified into a group of 13 subtypes, a set of disorders that affect connective tissues in the body. The most widespread type is Hypermobile EDS (hEDS), characterised by hypermobility of the joints and fragile skin that bruises easily or is overly stretchy. The more severe Vascular EDS (vEDS) impacts the fragile internal blood vessels and can cause extreme bleeding or organ problems due to incredibly thin skin offering little protection. The symptoms can lead to further complications such as breaks and dislocations, early-onset arthritis and, in the case of vEDS, ruptures of vital organs. EDS is primarily an inherited condition, more often than not via autosomal dominant inheritance, passed on via parent (one type, Kyphoscoliotic EDS, is inherited from a faulty gene from both parents). Family members will only ever inherit the same type of EDS as their parents.

Daily management of EDS requires an awareness and possible avoidance of activities and processes that could increase the risk of bodily harm, for example, playing certain high-intensity contact sports. Treatment addresses the symptoms through a variety of techniques. For vascular EDS especially, regular medical assessments are important to keep an eye on potential problems within the internal organs. Genetic counselling may help to process the onset of the condition, whilst cognitive behavioural therapy and talking therapies focus more on the pain an individual is experiencing. As with other conditions concerning joints and mobility, physiotherapy or occupational therapy can assist with improving the ease of daily activities.

Encephalitis

Whilst relatively uncommon, Encephalitis is incredibly serious and can pose a threat to life if urgent treatment is not obtained as soon as possible. It is an inflammation of the brain, most often caused by an infection directly impacting the brain. Herpes simplex virus is the most frequent cause, along with other common viruses such as measles, mumps, rubella and chickenpox. Another potential cause is a breakdown of the body's immune system which then erroneously turns and attacks the brain – this can be the result of infection, illness or even a vaccination. The first symptoms experienced are often those akin to having the flu, which can be coupled with a headache, drowsiness or feelings of confusion. The onset of symptoms for infectious encephalitis can happen within hours or days, sometimes resulting in a loss of consciousness; the onset of autoimmune encephalitis on the other hand tends to be slower and have many more symptoms such as altered behaviour, hallucinations or memory loss.

Possible treatment will vary depending on the symptoms. Steroid injections are administered to help fight encephalitis caused by issues with the immune system, along with immunoglobulin therapy for continued care. If a virus is discovered as the cause, antiviral medicine can be utilised. In rarer cases where the cause is discovered as a fungal or bacterial infection, a course of antibiotics is likely to be more suitable. The after-effects of encephalitis can be lengthy and complicated, even manifesting themselves years after the illness. When nerve cells in the brain are damaged, ongoing assessment and treatment is required to ensure recovery and rehabilitation is as successful as it can be. As the brain is unseen, this invisible illness can require a significant level of emotional support to overcome.

Endometriosis

Endometriosis is a long-term, chronic, and debilitating condition that affects females of any age (a handful of rare cases have been reported in males). The womb, or uterus, is lined with cells that build up and break down over the course of a cycle, leaving the body as a period. Endometriosis is caused when cells similar to this grow in other areas of the body, following the same menstrual cycle but are unable to leave the body – instead causing inflammation and pain. The condition often runs in families and genes are believed to play a part in the cause. Other theories suggest that endometriosis is a result of problems with the immune system, retrograde menstruation (where menstrual blood flows in the wrong direction) or exacerbated from previous surgery scars.

Symptoms can vary from female to female and indeed some with the condition may experience no symptoms at all. Periods may be particularly heavy and many of the common symptoms are experienced during this time, including tummy or pelvic pain, and gut or bowel problems such as constipation, diarrhoea or pain when urinating or defecating. Endometriosis can also cause pain during intercourse, infertility and an increased risk of mental health problems due to the isolating nature of the condition.

Common over-the-counter painkillers such as paracetamol and ibuprofen can help treat the pain. Surgery is an option, cutting away and removing areas of built up scar tissue. A hysterectomy – removal of the womb – may be deemed in severe cases.

Epilepsy

Epilepsy is a relatively common neurological disorder, affected around 1 in 100 people in the UK. The onset of symptoms usually happens either during childhood or when a person reaches over the age of 65. There is no definitive cause of epilepsy; it is believed that genetics may play a part as around a third of those with the condition also have a family member who has it. Another likelihood is previous damage to the brain, either from a head injury, stroke, infection or tumour.

A diagnosis is generally only made after an individual has had at least two seizures. Depending on which part of the brain the abnormal electrical activity is situated, seizures can result in different symptoms. Focal or partial seizures are caused by activity in one area of the brain. Generalised seizures involve all areas and include absence seizures, tonic, atonic, clonic, myoclonic and tonic-clonic seizures, the latter of which are considered to be the most severe. The main symptoms of epilepsy are the well-recognised uncontrollable jerky movements – sometimes leading to temporary unconsciousness – stiffening of muscles or a loss of control, staring blankly into space or peculiar sensations within the body. Seizures can seemingly happen quite randomly but can also be brought on as a result of triggers including stress, medication, alcohol or tiredness. Flashing lights are also a potential trigger, although this tends to be more uncommon that one might believe.

The main treatment is medication. In cases where only one specific section of the brain is responsible, targeted surgery may be an option. Adopting a specific keto diet can also help to keep the symptoms under control.

Fetal Alcohol Spectrum Disorders

Drinking alcohol during pregnancy can increase the risk of health problems in the baby, collectively known as Fetal Alcohol Spectrum Disorders (FASDs). Alcohol travels in the mother's blood, passing through the placenta and to the fetus, causing developmental damage. A fetus is unable to process alcohol like an adult is and all FASDs are entirely avoidable if the mother completely avoids alcohol during her pregnancy. Prenatal exposure to alcohol can cause 3 main disorders – Fetal Alcohol Syndrome (FAS), Alcohol-Related Birth Defects (ARBD) and Alcohol-Related Neurodevelopmental Disorder (ARND) – and it is possible to have more than one at the same time.

The symptoms of FAS are the most significant, causing physical abnormalities – characteristically a thin upper lip, horizontal eyes and a smooth area between the lip and nose, as well as a smaller head, and stunted growth. ARBD results in organ and bone formation and functionality problems, whilst ARND directly affects the brain and central nervous system resulting in behavioural or learning difficulties. All disorders can bring about further problems with hearing and vision and issues with focus and attention. FASDs are one of the leading, non-genetic causes of learning disabilities.

The key to management and support of the disorders is early diagnosis and intervention. It is impossible to overturn the physical damage done pre-birth and a programme of relevant educational and behavioural development strategies and treatments are likely to be required.

Fibromyalgia

Due to its symptoms being remarkably similar to a number of other conditions, Fibromyalgia is regularly misunderstood and misdiagnosed. As a chronic illness, it's not clear what causes fibromyalgia but a genetic predisposition is believed to be significant. Triggers such as trauma, injury or surgery can aggravate the onset of symptoms, as can lifestyle situations such as grief, abuse or family breakdowns. Pain is the predominant symptom of fibromyalgia, either in specific areas or throughout the body. Increased sensitivity can mean that the pain is felt more strongly (known as hyperalgesia) or as a result of something that would not usually cause pain to anyone else (allodynia). Muscles may feel stiff or spasm. Other common symptoms include headaches and fatigue, particularly because it may prevent an individual from obtaining deep, restorative sleep. There is also a link between fibromyalgia and cognition and mental health, due to low levels of specific hormones – this can lead to depression and anxiety. Treatment is aimed at easing symptoms and improving quality of life, since there is no known cure at present; more often than not a range of treatments will be explored to target the variety of symptoms. Medication such as painkillers, anticonvulsants and antipsychotics may lessen the physical indicators while antidepressants and sleeping pills can target the mental strains. A combination of rheumatological, neurological and psychological treatments can address the wide range of issues, utilising therapies such as hydrotherapy and tailored exercises combined with cognitive behavioural therapy, psychotherapy or relaxation techniques. For non-medical treatments, alternative therapies including acupuncture, aromatherapy and regular massage may provide some relief from daily chronic pain.

Food Allergies

Food Allergies are caused when the antibodies produced by the body's immune system incorrectly identify certain proteins in food and considers them a threat, releasing chemicals and prompting an allergic reaction. The most common antibody is immunoglobulin (IgE) which causes a chemical called histamine to be released – this is responsible for causing many of the typical allergy symptoms in particular areas of the body, known as IgE-mediated food allergies. There are also non-IgE-mediated food allergies caused by other cells.

Food allergies affect a huge number of people, children and adults alike, and there is a growing number, likely due in part to a changing diet. There are eight core foods that trigger almost all food allergies: peanuts, tree nuts, cow's milk, eggs, soy, wheat, fish and shellfish. Some people may also have reactions not to the food itself but rather the additives used in it such as sulphites and benzoates. Symptoms of an allergic reaction develop very quickly within a few minutes of consuming the food. A standard reaction may cause a tingling sensation within the mouth, swelling around the mouth, face or throat leading to problems with swallowing. The skin may turn itchy or red (with or without a rash) and it may be coupled with nausea, vomiting and dizziness. In the worst case it might trigger an anaphylactic shock in which symptoms worsen very quickly and can be deadly if immediate medical help is not obtained.

For known allergies, avoidance of the foods is the best way to manage the condition, but it is not always possible. Antihistamines are used to control most moderate allergies and in the case of potential anaphylaxis, adrenaline is administered via an auto-injector such as an EpiPen.

Friedreich's Ataxia

Ataxia (meaning a 'lack of control') is a term used to describe a group of disorders affecting coordination, balance, speech and swallowing. The conditions are usually a result of damage to the cerebellar, a part of the brain that controls balance and coordination. The most common type is Friedreich's ataxia (FRDA); others include Ataxia-telangiectasia (AT), Spinocerebellar ataxias (SCAs) and Episodic ataxia. Friedreich's ataxia is a rare hereditary disorder caused by a faulty autosomal recessive gene called FXN, carried down from both the mother and father. Also known as spinocerebellar degeneration, symptoms tend to manifest around the age of 10-15 and before the age of 25. Neurological symptoms include impaired balance, muscle weakness and loss of expected reflexes. Muscles in the heart can thicken and cause damage (cardiomyopathy) leading to shortness of breath and arrhythmias. Vision and hearing can be impacted, and speech may become slow and slurred or erratic. Generally, the use of a wheelchair is required approximately 10-20 years after the onset of the condition. As a result, people with Friedreich's ataxia tend to have a shorter life expectancy.

Given that ataxia affects multiple areas, a multidisciplinary team usually review and produce a unique care plan. Various therapies can assist with daily activities whilst orthopaedic interventions such as prostheses and wheelchairs aim to keep the individual as active as possible. Medication helps to control heart problems and some sight and hearing issues. Living with the condition can put a huge strain on mental health so treatments for depression or anxiety disorders may also be recommended, as well as genetic counselling in consideration of the condition being hereditary.

Hereditary Fructose Intolerance

Fructose is the natural sugar present within fruit, one of three monosaccharides along with glucose and galactose. It can also be found in honey, some root vegetables and in processed foods that contain added sugars. An enzyme called aldolase B is responsible for the transfer of breaking fructose down into energy; Heredity Fructose Intolerance (HFI) prevents this process from happening efficiently and instead when fructose is ingested, results in a toxic accumulation of fructose-1-phosphate which can eventually cause damage to the cells in the liver. A purely heredity condition, HFI is caused by mutations in the autosomal recessive gene ALDOB, passed down via both parents. Symptoms of HFI can be spotted in babies who are not feeding particularly well and when introduced to fruits and vegetables for the first time, may result in nausea, vomiting, sweating or extreme lethargy. It can also present as jaundice and if not picked up early, trigger convulsions or loss of consciousness. Treatment comes through a complete avoidance of fructose in the diet as well as sucrose and sorbitol too. A dietician will be able to advise what foods are suitable as an alternative, such as glucose or other sugars. Where the liver has been extremely irreparably damaged to the point it is potentially life-threatening, a liver transplant is an option, but this is rare in the standard treatment of HFI.

Fructose Malabsorption

Previously known as dietary fructose intolerance (and unrelated to heredity fructose intolerance), Fructose Malabsorption arises when certain cells are unable to effectively break down fructose. As a result, a build-up of fructose can develop in the large intestine causing issues in the gut. There are a number of potential causes including excessive consumption of processed or refined food, a disparity in the levels of healthy and non-healthy bacteria within the gut and increased stress levels. It is also believed that a change in diet and rise in the consumption of fructose in many people's daily food intake has resulted in an increase of cases of fructose malabsorption.

Often misdiagnosed as IBS as it shares similar symptoms, characteristics of fructose malabsorption include gastrointestinal problems such as bloating, nausea, flatulence, diarrhoea and abdominal pain. Some people may also be at an increased risk of developing mental health problems since there has been a link found between fructose malabsorption and lower levels of an amino acid called tryptophan, which is associated with producing serotonin to stabilise mood.

Those with pre-existing gut disorders are more likely to also have fructose malabsorption and a restricted diet is best to avoid a flareup of symptoms. Not only can it be found in most fruits, high levels of fructose are also present in vegetables such as broccoli, peas and leeks, many desserts and sweet treats that contain fructose sweeteners and some natural sweeteners such as honey and agave syrup. In some cases, antibiotics or probiotics may be prescribed to aid bacterial overgrowth in the small intestine.

Hashimoto's Thyroiditis

Affecting significantly more women than men and particularly those between the ages of 30 and 50, Hashimoto's Thyroiditis is an autoimmune disease that causes damage to the thyroid gland. Located in the bottom of the neck, the thyroid gland produces hormones that control many of the body's functions, particularly the metabolic process. The cause is unclear though a combination of genetics, bacterial or viral infection and age is likely to be involved. Antibodies from the immune system mistakenly attack the thyroid gland, causing damage and an inability to produce thyroid hormone which can lead to hypothyroidism (an underactive thyroid). In turn this can bring on symptoms such as fatigue, dry skin and weight gain. In addition, as the disease tends to develop over many years, there may be muscle weakness or joint pain, hair loss, brittle nails, memory lapses or irregular menstrual bleeding. The swelling and constant stimulation of the thyroid can produce a goitre, or lump, in the throat. Other thyroiditis types can also cause a swelling of the thyroid gland – De Quervain's thyroiditis, postpartum thyroiditis, silent thyroiditis, drug-induced or radiation-induced thyroiditis or acute or infectious thyroiditis.

Treatment is usually in the form of medication which will need to be taken for the remainder of a lifetime. Taken orally, Levothyroxine is a synthetic thyroid hormone which can balance and restore the correct hormone levels. Usually it can reverse the effects of hypothyroidism and relieve many of the associated symptoms. Thyroid surgery may be appropriate to exclusively treat a goitre that is impacting the ability to consume or drink – depending on the underlying cause, removal of a part or all of the thyroid gland is an option.

HIV and AIDS

HIV, human immunodeficiency virus, impacts the cells in the body's immune system, decreasing its strength and ability in fighting off disease and infections. HIV can be transmitted between people via bodily fluids and certain groups are at higher risk of transmitting and being infected: Black African people, men who have sex with other men and injection drug users who may engage in risky actions such as sharing syringes or needles. The initial symptoms of HIV is known as seroconversion illness, a short fever, rash or sore throat not dissimilar to flu symptoms, but the virus will carry on causing undetected harm for many years – meaning that it can be difficult to diagnose. When left untreated, HIV causes significant damage to the immune system and can develop into a number of infections and illnesses known by the term Acquired Immune

Deficiency Syndrome, or AIDS. Whilst the term AIDS is not regularly used any longer (instead referred to as late-stage HIV), it was prevalent in the 1980s when HIV was identified. If late-stage HIV is developed then it can cause unexplained, rapid weight loss, recurring night sweats, swelling of the lymph glands, extended bouts of diarrhoea or serious, potentially life-threatening infections such as tuberculosis, pneumonia or cancer.

Post-exposure prophylaxis (PEP) is an emergency medicine that can potentially eliminate the chance of being infected with HIV, providing it is taken within approximately 24-72 hours of exposure. The main form of treatment are antiretroviral tablets, taken daily to stop the virus from being able to replicate. As HIV can easily develop resistance, a combination of various tablets is best to increase their impact.

Hyperhidrosis

It is not uncommon for everyone to sweat from time to time, a natural cooling process for the body in response to, for example, heat, stress or strenuous exercise. Hyperhidrosis is a form of extreme sweating in relation to no obvious reason. The cause is unclear – for some it may be the standard triggers that cause most people to sweat, for others it could be other related endocrine or neurological conditions.

Symptoms of hyperhidrosis usually manifest in the places one might expect to sweat – the face, underarms (axillary hyperhidrosis), or the hands and feet (palmoplantar hyperhidrosis). The sweating itself is usually harmless and primarily results in frustration and potential embarrassment for the individual. It can lead to dislike or avoidance of certain professional or social situations, impact relationships and sometimes increase the risk of mood disorders.

There are a number of treatment options depending on which parts of the body are impacted. The initial treatment recommendation is an antiperspirant containing aluminium chloride, typically available over the counter, and if that shows no improvement, a prescription strength antiperspirant containing the stronger aluminium chloride hexahydrate. Iontophoresis is a process that utilises ionised tap water to transfer low voltage electrical currents through the skin of the affected area (usually hands or feet). Anticholinergics are oral medications taken to ease sweating and techniques using Botox, microwave energy and lasers can be utilised to kill the sweat glands on a permanent basis. In extreme cases surgery can even be an option, using a procedure called a thoracic sympathectomy.

Hypoglycaemia

Most cases of Hypoglycaemia (low blood sugar level) are recorded in people who have diabetes, however there are some rare cases of non-diabetic hypoglycaemia. There are two main types: reactive hypoglycaemia, which occurs within a few hours of eating a large meal rich in carbohydrate, and fasting hypoglycaemia (nesidioblastosis) which is extremely rare and usually linked with a more serious condition. Reactive hypoglycaemia means that the body is unable to stabilise blood sugar levels or it generates too much insulin. Whilst uncommon, this can increase the risk of becoming diabetic. Fasting hypoglycaemia may be caused when the liver or kidneys have been impacted, such as using certain medication or taking in extreme levels of alcohol. It has also been linked to some eating disorders, pregnancy and post-surgical complications in the stomach region (known as dumping syndrome). The onset of hypoglycaemic indicators tends to happen relatively quickly, feeling shaky, lightheaded or dizzy, skin feeling sweaty or clammy, a fast heartbeat and feelings of intense hunger. Emotions can be anxious or confused or irritable. At worst, seizures may occur and lead to the individual collapsing or losing consciousness.

Immediate treatment is to eat or drink something containing sugar, such as a biscuit, a few sweets or a carbonated drink, before checking the blood sugar level to ensure it is at the correct level and the symptoms have eased. In cases of more serious or and regular hypoglycaemia, the individual may be required to carry glucose in the form of tablets or an injection and regularly monitor their symptoms.

Inclusion Body Myositis

Inclusion Body Myositis (IBM) is a progressive disorder that causes weakness and inflammation in the muscles. Unlike the other types of myositis, polymyositis and dermatomyositis, it is seen more often in men than women and symptoms do not generally emerge until around the age of 50 and beyond, when they gradually worsen over years. The cause of IBM is unclear; it is thought that either inflammation caused by a virus damages the muscles, or it can be classified as a degenerative disease. There is evidence that some people are at a higher risk due to a genetic predisposition, but it is generally not considered hereditary.

With IBM, the muscles that tend to be most affected are the quadriceps (thighs), followed by the forearms and then wrists and fingers. The muscles can feel weak, tender and painful. Sometimes the facial and throat muscles can also be impacted, leading to mild difficulties with swallowing (dysphagia). As the condition progresses it is likely that support will be required with some daily activities such as climbing stairs, getting up from a chair or gripping objects. In some cases, a wheelchair may be needed when leg muscle strength and function has deteriorated. Mood disorders, particularly depression, is often seen in conjunction and can even be an indicator before the point of IBM diagnosis.

There is no treatment or effective therapy for IBM; some specialists suggest immunosuppressant treatments whilst others recommend immunoglobulin infusions – there is no evidence that either provide long-term benefits. Instead a combination of exercise and physiotherapy treatment aims to develop and maintain muscle strength in order to lessen the impact on daily activities.

Interstitial Cystitis

Significantly more common in women than men, symptoms of Interstitial Cystitis are generally first displayed in individuals in their 30's and 40's. Sometimes also referred to as Bladder Pain Syndrome (BPS), the condition directly affects the bladder but can have a huge range of symptoms with varying degrees of severity, making it hard to diagnose. There is usually no evidence of infection within the bladder, but damage to the lining of the organ can result in inflammation, ulceration or scarring. Alternative causes may an allergic reaction or issues with the pelvic floor muscles.

Damage within the bladder can lead to irritation of the muscles and nerves within it, stemming intense pain in the pelvic region. The urge to urinate can be sudden and strong, requiring trips to the toilet more frequently and especially during the night. The pain may be episodic, lasting for set phases of weeks or months, or for women may be triggered and worsened during periods.

Before medication, it may be possible to reduce pain caused by interstitial cystitis through lifestyle alterations; wearing looser clothing to prevent any additional pressure, reducing stress as much as possible, stopping smoking, drinking alcohol or eating certain foods (tomatoes or citrus fruits, for example) and applying a routine to toilet breaks to prevent the bladder from reaching capacity. If symptoms show no improvement then medication can be prescribed to help soothe irritation in the bladder, control spasms and help repair the inner tissues. With ongoing pain, a urologist may recommend certain procedures such as bladder stretching to increase capacity or neurostimulation to target the nerves and reduce pain.

Irritable Bowel Syndrome

Relatively widespread and known as IBS, Irritable Bowel Syndrome is a lifelong condition that causes distress to the body's digestive system. Possible causes are an oversensitive immune system or abnormalities in the colon, or a previous bacterial or viral infection. Whilst there is no set established cause, known triggers that worsen the symptoms include stress, hormones (particularly as women are more likely to experience issues around the time of their period) or certain foods or beverages. Symptoms can range from mild to severe, causing mild annoyance or severe disruption to daily activities. They include diarrhoea and constipation, abdominal pain and bloating – for which a bowel movement usually provides some relief. Due to the impact of IBS, it can be intricately linked to mood disorders such as depression and anxiety.

Depending on individual symptoms, a series of lifestyle and diet choices are the best way to manage IBS. Reducing the amount of caffeinated, alcoholic or carbonated drinks can help, as can cooking fresh, wholesome meals with minimal processed or fatty foods. Certain foods, such as porridge oats or pulses, are linked with the reduction of bloating, as opposed to some vegetables which are harder to digest. A pharmacist may recommend over-the-counter medication to relieve some of the symptoms; probiotics for bloating, loperamide for diarrhoea or laxatives to reduce constipation. Exercising regularly, using progressive relaxation techniques and engaging in stress-reducing activities may also ease pain and reduce symptoms.

Kennedy's Disease

Kennedy's Disease has a number of other names, but most common is Spinal and Bulbar Muscular Atrophy (SBMA). It is a rare progressive neuro-muscular condition that is caused by a genetic mutation. Generally, symptoms do not emerge until adulthood amid the ages of 30 to 50 and develop almost exclusively in men. Women can carry the faulty gene but rarely display any symptoms. Due to the symptoms being comparable to those of other conditions a misdiagnosis is possible, and a DNA blood test is the only method to determine the presence of the disease.

Weakness and wastage of the muscles is a key indicator, especially in the arms or legs. This may be coupled with muscular pain, cramps, tremors, twitches or a rippling sensation (fasciculations). The bulbar muscles which control the throat and its various functions can also be impacted, affecting the ability to talk or swallow food (dysphagia). Fatigue is also relatively common, and some individuals experience an enlargement of the glands in the breast area (gynecomastia).

Similar to motor neurone conditions, there is currently no evident cure for Kennedy's disease; instead, support is aimed at management of the symptoms. Ongoing physical and occupational therapy can identify adaptations such as walking aids or wheelchairs. Speech therapy may be suitable for those with worsening dysphagia whilst surgery is sometimes an option for those with gynecomastia. Depending on the symptoms and severity, certain types of medication may prove successful in reducing them.

Lactose Intolerance

Lactose is a sugar found mainly in milk, but also dairy products or foods made with milk derivatives. An enzyme called lactase is produced by the body's digestive system to break down the lactose so it can be absorbed. Unlike a milk allergy, which is a reaction to the proteins in milk, having a lactose intolerance means that the body does not make enough lactase and as a result the lactose is broken down by bacteria in the large intestine instead, causing unwelcome symptoms. There are various types of lactase deficiency – primary (caused by inherited faulty genes), secondary (resulting from problems with the small intestine), congenital (rare but seen in some new-born babies) and developmental (found in premature babies). Consuming dairy products that contain lactose will bring on the symptoms, usually around 1-2 hours after consumption. For some individuals, the symptoms can be mild or uncomfortable, such as flatulence or bloating, but for others they can be painful and disruptive. Abdominal pain can be severe, combined with nausea, vomiting or diarrhoea.

If lactose intolerance is only temporary (for example, due to a bout of gastroenteritis) then the symptoms should disappear after a short time. For long-term intolerance, the best control of the condition is to completely cut out all lactose from the diet. Lactose-free milk (such as oat, almond or soya milk) and dairy products, including yoghurt and cheese, are becoming readily available. To ensure the body is receiving enough calcium, vital for bone and teeth health, supplements may need to be taken. Lactase substitutes are also an option in potentially reducing symptoms.

Lupus

Systemic Lupus Erythematosus (SLE), more widely known as Lupus, is a disease caused by the body's immune system producing an excess of antibodies which mistakenly attack tissues throughout the body, resulting in inflammation and damage to various organs. Its cause is believed to be a combination of genetics and environmental factors – certain medication, previous infections and even exposure to sunlight are thought to be potential triggers. It tends to affect more women than men and is usually diagnosed around the age of 15 – 55.

Cases of lupus can result in multiple different symptoms, making it hard to diagnose. The main indicators are pain in the joint or muscles and intense tiredness which does not ease with rest or sleep. A distinctive rash resembling butterfly wings may also appear across the cheeks and nose; lupus, meaning 'wolf', gets its name from this rash as it was thought to bear a resemblance the bite of a wolf. Other symptoms include headaches, fever, recurrent mouth ulcers, possible hair loss, increased light sensitivity and Raynaud's syndrome. Depending on the severity of the condition for the individual, symptoms may come and go in flare ups, or be regular and constant. Extreme damage to the kidneys or lungs may even be life-threatening. Given the inflammatory nature of the disease, non-steroidal anti-inflammatory (NSAIDs) medication is generally a first line of treatment. Hydroxychloroquine, a type of anti-malarial drug, can help to ease both chronic fatigue and joint pain, as well as ease skin conditions. For more serious cases, a combination of corticosteroids and immunosuppressants are generally used to suppress the inflammation and prevent further organ damage.

Lyme Disease

Lyme Disease (or Lyme borreliosis) is one of several tick-borne diseases, though by far the most common. Ticks are tiny arachnids, not dissimilar to a small spider, that live in long grass of parks or gardens. They attach themselves to skin in order to feed on the blood of humans or animals. Whilst the majority of tick bites are harmless, a small number of ticks carry a bacterium which can be transferred to a human through a bite and cause an infection, Lyme disease.

Initial symptoms tend to be headaches and aches in the muscles or joints, combined with fatigue, energy loss or a high temperature. From the point of the bite, these symptoms typically appear within 4 weeks, but it can be a few months. Around three quarters of people will also develop a characteristic painless red, circular rash (called erythema migrans) around the point of the bite. It can look a little like a bullseye on a dartboard and is often key to a diagnosis as many of the main symptoms can easily be confused with those of other conditions. Left untreated, symptoms can develop and worsen over a number of years, including heart palpitations, extreme tiredness, numbness or difficulty moving the limbs.

Early treatment is paramount in curing Lyme disease. A course of antibiotics is predominantly the primary action, which may need to be taken for around a month. In more severe cases the antibiotics may be injected under hospital treatment. It can take a number of months for symptoms to completely ease and disappear, but they do generally cease for most people.

Metabolic Syndrome

Diabetes, high blood pressure and obesity are all conditions in their own right; Metabolic Syndrome is the combination of all three. It affects approximately a third of all adults over the age of 50 and the causes are linked predominantly with inactivity and obesity. So too is insulin resistance, a condition that prevents glucose from entering the relevant cells in the body and therefore increases sugar levels in the blood. Insulin resistance is linked with type 2 diabetes indeed the biggest risk factor of metabolic syndrome is the increased chances of developing that condition too. You are more likely to develop metabolic syndrome if you have had other conditions including polycystic ovary syndrome (PCOS), non-alcoholic fatty liver disease (NAFLD), sleep apnoea or gestational diabetes during pregnancy.

The symptoms are typically a large waist circumference (94cm or more in European men and 80cm plus in European women), high blood pressure (hypertension) and high triglyceride or cholesterol levels. There may also be swelling or irritation of certain body tissues and a tendency to develop blood clots.

Significant lifestyle changes are required to avoid or overturn the effects of metabolic syndrome. Adopting a healthy lifestyle by losing weight, eating a nutritious, varied diet and doing regular exercise are key, as is cutting back on drinking alcohol or smoking cigarettes. Specific medication can be given for certain issues such as high blood pressure or high cholesterol levels.

Migraines

Unlike a mild headache that most people will have experienced at some point, a Migraine is a much more complex condition that as well as a severe headache, can include a number of other symptoms. Migraines affect significantly more women than men and have usually started by the early adult years. Whilst the cause is unknown, they are generally considered to be hereditary and commonly triggered by situations such as stress, food or sleep deprivation and in women, hormonal shifts. There are numerous types of migraine but the most prominent is known as a migraine without aura – there are no obvious triggers or warning signs before the onset of the symptoms, which last anywhere between 4 hours and a few days and the frequency can be as little as once a year or as regularly as a few times a week. Less frequent is a migraine with aura, preceded with certain neurological warning signals such as flashing lights, blind spots, colours, tunnel vision or vertigo. For migraines to be considered chronic they must occur at least 15 times per month. Some individuals experience a four-stage process: prodrome (subtle physical or mood alterations), aura (visual disturbances), attack (throbbing or pulsing pain, vomiting or sensitivity to light, sounds and smells) and post-drome (feelings of exhaustion or elation).

The first step to recognising and diagnosing migraines is documenting the severity, frequency and possible triggers. This may help to avoid certain situations or provide an increased awareness of when a migraine could be likely. Over-the-counter painkillers such as paracetamol and ibuprofen, or prescribed medication including triptans or anti-emetics can be effective in lessening the symptoms once they occur.

Multiple Chemical Sensitivity

There is some debate about whether Multiple Chemical Sensitivity (MCS) can be clinically classified as an illness, but with multiple triggers and a wide range of symptoms, it can have a hugely detrimental impact on those individuals who have it. It can develop at any age and essentially the immune system is unable to process harmful toxins that enter the body. It is thought that the internal detoxification systems stop being productive as a result of either exposure to one particular toxin or can develop over time post-infection or viral illness. Consequently, individuals are over-sensitive to numerous chemicals found in everyday items, such as household cleaning solutions, beauty products and perfumes or common pesticides, and symptoms are triggered even after extremely low exposure to these. It is possible to develop sensitivities to certain foods, requiring a complete change of diet, or even electromagnetic fields found in televisions, computers or telephones. Sometimes an individual may not have any idea what their trigger is since irritants can also be airborne and untraceable. Symptoms can be hugely varied dependent on the cause and are similar to those of any allergic reactions: headaches, muscular pain, rashes on the skin, nausea and exhaustion. They can occur soon after exposure to the chemical or a few hours later. There are no proven treatments for MCS. When the chemical trigger is known, care can be taken to avoid the area or specific products that contain it. Opting for 'environmentally friendly' and natural products can reduce the presence of potential chemical triggers. Since MCS can be isolating and hard to manage, antidepressants or sleeping aids may be recommended to reduce the likelihood of additional mood disorders.

Multiple Sclerosis

Affecting the body's central nervous system, Multiple Sclerosis (MS) is a lifelong condition which generally causes significant disability for the individual. Specifically, the layer of myelin that surrounds and protects the nerves is mistakenly attacked by the immune system, resulting in inflammation. The impact of this damage to the myelin sheath (sclerosis) causes disruption to the messages travelling between the body and brain, which leads to the symptoms of MS. It impacts far more women than men, with diagnoses generally being made between the ages of 20 and 40. Individual genetics increase the chance of developing the condition, as does obesity (particularly in the teenage years), smoking and certain viral infections. It is also thought that a deficiency in vitamin D from sunlight increase a person's risk.

Debilitating fatigue is one of the main symptoms of MS, along with difficulties walking caused by issues with balance or pain, weakness or numbness in the lower limbs. Individuals may also experience problems with vision (optic neuritis), thinking and memory, speech or swallowing, bladder or bowel issues or mood disorders such as anxiety or depression. Like many other illnesses, the symptoms of MS can be unpredictable and different for everyone, with relapses and remissions or a gradual deterioration over time. As such, treatment is usually considered by a multidisciplinary team of medical professionals. A flare-up of symptoms may be treated with a course of steroid tablets or injections, whilst disease-modifying therapies (DMTs) are used to lessen the frequency of relapses and potentially diminish the speed of symptoms worsening.

Multiple System Atrophy

A relatively rare condition, Multiple System Atrophy (MSA) is often cited as having similar attributes to Parkinson's disease. Both are progressive neurological disorders but there are some unique symptoms to MSA, and it is typically diagnosed at an earlier age, around the early 50s. At present there are no established causes of MSA; it is not hereditary and there are no known environmental factors – it is believed that the condition is sporadic and can affect anyone. The symptoms are caused by an accumulation of alpha-synuclein, a type of protein found in the brain cells, which causes damage to various but specific parts of the brain. This leads to wide-ranging issues that impact the autonomic nervous system, including urinary processes, blood pressure and movement of muscles throughout the body.

For many, the primary symptoms of MSA are feelings of dizziness or fainting after standing up, due to postural hypertension (low blood pressure). Many people will experience bladder problems, such as being unable to urinate, needing to go more frequently or losing bladder control. Men commonly have erectile dysfunction. If the cerebellum section of the brain is damaged (known as cerebellar ataxia), it usually causes issues with co-ordination and balance. This can result in unsteadiness, bradykinesia (moving slowly) and stiffness in the muscles. Others may experience sleeping problems, noisy gasping or breathing and unpredictable emotional responses such as irrepressibly laughing or crying. It is not possible to cure MSA nor hinder the progression of the symptoms, rather provide long-term support and care as life expectancy is shortened to fewer than 10 years after diagnosis.

Myasthenia Gravis

Myasthenia Gravis is an autoimmune condition which results in the receptors between the nerves and muscles being wrongly attacked by antibodies in the immune system. It is thought that an enlarged thymus gland might be responsible for this, impacting communication signals and causing muscle weakness. Uncommon in children, diagnoses are predominantly made in women aged under the age of 40 but in men over the age of 60.

Onset of symptoms can be quite sudden and are usually first noticeable in the face and eyes – droopy eyelids (either one or both), possible double vision and weak facial muscles. If only the muscles around the eyes are impacted, it is known as ocular myasthenia. The weakness may spread to the jaw and throat resulting in difficulty swallowing (dysphagia), breathing or speaking. It can also affect the arms or legs, though more common in the upper body, making daily physical activities challenging. Sometimes specific triggers, including emotional stress, lack of sleep or medication, can increase the severity of the symptoms so avoidance of these where possible is recommended. Tablets of pyridostigmine are usually the first step to treatment; they can be taken frequently to assist communication between nerves and muscles. As an autoimmune condition, immunosuppressants are used to aid the immune system. Where the thymus gland is considered a potential cause, surgery to remove it can reduce the requirement for medication. In its most severe form, when respiratory muscles have been compromised and the individual is unable to breathe (myasthenic crisis), emergency treatments will be delivered in the form of a ventilator, plasmapheresis or intravenous immunoglobulin therapy.

Narcolepsy

Narcolepsy is a rare but relatively well-known lifelong disorder characterised by the unusual characteristic of suddenly falling asleep. Despite its symptoms, narcolepsy is not considered a sleep disorder but rather a central nervous system disorder. A chemical present in the brain, called hypocretin or orexin, is responsible for regulating sleep – narcolepsy can be caused when the immune system wrongly attacks the cells in the part of the brain that create hypocretin. It may also impact a protein named trib 2, found in the same area of the brain, responsible for producing hypocretin. However, some individuals diagnosed with narcolepsy do have normal levels of hypocretin, so it is likely not to be the sole cause. Increased risks come from faulty genes, major hormonal changes or significant stress, or as a result of a previous infection or identifiable underlying condition. Regular drowsiness or excessive daytime sleepiness (EDS) are usually the first visible signs of narcolepsy. Some individuals may have sudden sleep attacks, a period of uncontrollable sleep that may last anywhere between a few seconds or a few minutes. The symptoms of cataplexy are also fairly common – an involuntary, temporary loss of muscular control, usually triggered by a strong emotional response such as laughter or surprise. Further symptoms can include hallucinations, memory problems, restless sleep or temporary sleep paralysis. The adoption of good, healthy sleeping habits is paramount to managing narcolepsy. Medications that potentially prompt drowsiness should be avoided but stimulants may be prescribed to help keep the individual awake. Talking to others with the condition may help to process the experience of living with narcolepsy.

Osteoporosis

Osteoporosis means 'spongy bone' and, as the name suggests, it is a condition that causes weakened, fragile bones that have a greater risk of breaking due to low density. Far more women are affected than men, likely due to a reduction in oestrogen hormone after the menopause which speeds up the process of bone loss. A number of risk factors increase the chances of developing osteoporosis, including family history of the condition, a poor diet with heavy drinking or smoking, a lack of exercise or having a low body weight. Steroids are also known to reduce the absorption of calcium which is crucial for bone strength.

Having osteoporosis means that bones have a higher chance of breaking, particularly as a result of a seemingly minor accident, but there can be no visible symptoms until that happens. Using a bone density scan (DEXA), it is possible to diagnose osteopenia, having lower-than-average bone density – there is no guarantee of it developing into osteoporosis, but the process can be slowed. Commonly the wrist is one of the weakest areas of the body and can easily break, as can the hip bones, when used to help try and prevent a trip or fall. Spinal or vertebral crush fractures are also commonplace and can result in curvature of the spine or postural changes; they can easily be mistaken for symptoms of arthritis.

Fragility factures of bones due to osteoporosis take the same time to heal as a normal broken bone and are treated in the same manner using a cast (where possible). To slow down the loss of bone density there are various medications that can be taken, such as bisphosphonates or selective oestrogen receptor modulators (SERMs), combined with vitamin D and calcium supplements.

Overactive Thyroid Gland

Often referred to as hyperthyroidism or sometimes thyrotoxicosis, an Overactive Thyroid Gland results in the excessive production of thyroid hormones, triiodothyronine (T3) and thyroxine (T4). Significantly more women than men are diagnosed, usually between the ages of 20 and 40. An autoimmune condition called Graves' disease is the most common cause of an overactive thyroid gland. Nodules (small, usually benign lumps) on the thyroid may also be responsible, or excessive levels of iodine from certain types of medication.

Wide-ranging symptoms can incorporate fatigue and muscle weakness, breathlessness, increased appetite, anxiety, irritability, restlessness or unpredictable emotions. With an imbalance of T3 or T4, the body can enter a hypermetabolic state – some of the physical characteristics include heart palpitations, sweaty or overly warm skin, hives, hair loss or unexpected weight loss. An enlarged lump may appear in the throat, known as a goitre. Some individuals may only experience a few mild symptoms with little impact, whereas for others it can lead to additional complications with eye conditions, pregnancy issues or a life-threatening thyroid storm which requires emergency medical intervention. Fortunately, treatment is usually successful for an overactive thyroid. The initial steps are medication in the form of beta-blockers or antithyroid drugs to curb production of hormones. Effectiveness is not generally seen for a couple of months and a full course can be around 18 months – if the symptoms return then a single radioactive iodine treatment can be considered. This destroys the thyroid gland cells, preventing further undue production of hormones. In some cases, surgery to remove the thyroid gland completely can be an option.

Personality Disorders

Caused by a mix of genetics, environmental factors and early childhood life experience, Personality Disorders impact the way that a person relates to themselves and others through thoughts, feelings or behaviours. There are currently ten individual disorders which can be categorised into three main types – suspicious, emotional and impulsive, and anxious. Paranoid personality disorder is linked with feelings of paranoia, mistrust and seeing potential danger where others typically would not. The schizotypal personality disorder is characterised by distorted or eccentric behaviours and beliefs. Those with schizoid personality disorder may be withdrawn, choosing to spending time alone and without close relationship, whilst people with antisocial personality disorder find it hard to empathise with others and act aggressively or impulsively. The most common personality disorder is borderline personality disorder (BPD), associated with intense, unstable emotions, a fear of abandonment, impulsive actions and potentially suicidal thoughts or self-harming. Those diagnosed with histrionic personality disorder depend on being noticed and seeking approval from others, not too dissimilar to narcissistic personality disorder which embodies being seen as dismissive or unaware of others with seemingly high self-esteem. Avoidant personality disorder is linked to social anxiety and fears of rejection, whilst dependent personality disorder is an unhealthy need for reassurance from others. The drive for control and perfectionism is iconic of obsessive compulsive personality disorder (OCPD).

Treatment varies depending on the specific symptoms but is likely to include a range of talking therapies (counselling, CBT or DBT), medication and access to therapeutic communities.

Phobias

A type of anxiety disorder, Phobias are more than a dislike or dread of a specific object or situation, rather an extreme, overwhelming and unrealistic fear. A fear develops into a phobia when it is disproportionate to the potential danger involved and is likely to have a detrimental influence on the individual's daily life. It is not entirely evident why all phobias develop. Some, known as simple or specific phobias, are correlated to a negative childhood experience which caused intense stress or fear. They can also be learned responses from witnessing family members who have a similar phobia. Specific phobias include animals (commonly spiders, snakes or dogs), the natural world (such as water, heights or the dark), situational (including flying, drowning or claustrophobia, a fear of small spaces) and body-related sources such as blood, injections or choking.

Brain chemistry and genes are more likely to initiate complex phobias, such as agoraphobia (fear of open or outside spaces) or social phobia (fear of being in social situations). Exposure to the source of the phobia, or sometimes even the thought of it, can trigger feelings of anxiety and panic. In response to complex phobias, the body tends to release adrenaline, causing physical bodily reactions such as sweating, shaking or panic attacks.

Whilst avoidance of the source may be suitable for some to control the phobia, for others it can actually intensify the phobia. Talking therapies and the process of exposure therapy – from talking about the phobia, to seeing an image, to being put in the situation or confronted with the source itself – have proved effective in many cases. Practising relaxation techniques may assist with learning to manage the stress and anxiety caused by a phobia.

Polycystic Ovary Syndrome

Often referred to as PCOS, Polycystic Ovary Syndrome is caused by a reproductive hormone imbalance in women. Relatively common, affecting around a tenth of women, the ovaries are impacted and unable to produce or release an egg during the menstrual cycle. The majority of PCOS cases are seen in women who are obese, leading to the assumption that obesity may be an underlying cause of the syndrome. It is thought to be linked with increased insulin levels which result in the ovaries producing too much testosterone, amongst other androgens (male hormones). Genetics are also credited to playing a role. Part of the diagnosis is made using an ultrasound which reveals multiple growths on the ovaries – although unlike the name suggests, these are not cysts but rather innocuous, immature follicles.

Over half of those with PCOS display no symptoms and may only be diagnosed when issues arise with getting pregnant, due to irregular or a complete lack of ovulation. Common characteristics of the syndrome include menstrual disorders, such as erratic periods or amenorrhea (a lack of periods for at least 3 consecutive months). An increased level of male hormones can prompt weight gain or excess hair growth around the face, back or chest, or hair loss from the head.

For women who are obese, weight loss through lifestyle changes is key to improving some of the symptoms of PCOS. Where periods are absent, the contraceptive pill or progestogen tablets can be used to promote onset and regulation. For women who are looking to get pregnant, medication called clomifene is used to stimulate ovulation, and in some cases a surgical procedure called laparoscopic ovarian drilling (LOD) may assist with infertility.

Polymyositis

One of the more common types of myositis, Polymyositis predominantly affects the muscles, joints or connective tissues of the neck, shoulders, hips and thigh muscles. Less common in men, diagnosis is mostly made between the ages of 30 and 60 but it is not apparent what causes polymyositis. The main line of thinking considers it an autoimmune disease, but it could also be as a result of a virus, infection or faulty immune system. Muscular weakness and pain are the main features of the condition, caused by vasculitis (swollen blood vessels). Due to the location of the muscles that are habitually impacted, individuals will find it difficult to sit up or stand up, particularly after a stumble or fall. It can also cause problems with holding the weight of the head or more acute issues with swallowing food. Some people may show symptoms of Raynaud's phenomenon, an intense reaction to the cold which can result in a spasm within the blood vessels. As the condition can be debilitating, people are also more likely to suffer from low mood and depression. Diagnosis can be confirmed through blood tests, electromyography (EMG) examinations or a muscle biopsy to confirm cell damage.

As a chronic illness there are a few different therapies that can be considered to help ease the problems associated with polymyositis. Physical exercise combined with physiotherapy is recommended to help restore and maintain muscle strength. Immunosuppressants or corticosteroids, both types of medication, work to minimise muscular swelling and associated pain. More rarely intravenous immunoglobulin provides a dose of antibodies from healthy blood to prevent further attack from the immune system.

Post-Traumatic Stress Disorder

Often referred to by the acronym PTSD, Post-Traumatic Stress Disorder was first diagnosed in war veterans, originally known as 'shell shock'. Triggered by a traumatic event, it is an anxiety disorder that can cause the individual to relive their horrific experience. Such situations may be being assaulted or abused, being involved in a car crash, natural disaster, or violent crime, witnessing a distressing situation happening to another person. Exposure to ongoing trauma, for example due to a job, increases the chances of developing PTSD, and it can rise if there is no support network or there are further causes of stress at the time.

The main symptoms include flashbacks or nightmares abouts the event, with physical reactions such as sweating or pain. It can cause panic, hypervigilance, irritability, sleeping problems or reckless behaviour. Depending on the cause, it can leave an individual with trust issues or feelings of being unsafe or alone, or self-blame, guilt or frustration. Complex post-traumatic stress disorder (CPTSD) can be characterised by experiencing symptoms of PTSD as well as additional emotional difficulties such as dissociation, relationship problems, or physical indicators, including stomach or chest pains and headaches.

Talking therapies, including counselling, group therapy (relevant to the trauma), trauma-focused cognitive behavioural therapy (TF-CBT) or dialectal behaviour therapy (DBT) have been found to be successful improving the symptoms of PTSD. Antidepressants might also be an option, particularly paroxetine or sertraline. CPTSD may be treated with a process called eye movement desensitisation and reprocessing (EMDR).

Primary Immunodeficiency Disorders

Primary Immunodeficiency is a group of over 300 rare disorders that directly impact the immune system, the body's natural defence against infection. They are caused by inherited faulty genes, so most individuals are born either without elements of the immune system, or certain parts that are faulty. They can usually be diagnosed fairly early on in a baby's life and the impact of primary immunodeficiency disorders (PIDs) can be significant with frequent and prolonged periods of illness.

The common characteristics of PIDs are persistent or recurring infections that are not always cured as effectively by conventional treatments. Certain infections are more commonplace, such as skin, ear or sinus infections, bronchitis or pneumonia. Depending on the type of PID, one might have digestion issues or blood disorders or conditions that impact normal development. Some may also develop infections that are considered unusual or rare. The acronym SPURR is useful for categorising potential PIDs: 'Severe, Persistent, Unusual, Recurrent infections, which Run in the family.'

Good hygiene, keeping active, embracing a healthy lifestyle and controlling stress levels are all positive steps to averting potential infections. In the event of an infection, a course of antibiotics is the most productive treatment. Immunoglobulin replacement therapy or bone marrow transplantation are the two main forms of treatment recommended by immunologists to give the body a boost of healthy white blood cells responsible for combating infection. If a person with a PID is considering having a family, genetic counselling can be helpful to process the implications of them being hereditary, and gene therapy may also be considered.

Prosopagnosia

Also called face blindness, Prosopagnosia is a peculiar impairment which results in the individual not being able to identify faces of other people. Developmental prosopagnosia is a condition that emerges from birth, thought to be linked to genetics. Acquired prosopagnosia on the other hand is significantly rarer and develops as a result of damage to the brain. The difficulty in diagnosing developmental prosopagnosia in particular is that the individual is unlikely to realise anything is untoward as they have never known any different. They will likely struggle to recognise faces that they have previously seen, regardless of whether that person is well known to them or not – in some cases an individual may not even recognise their own family members, closest friends or indeed themselves in photos or in the mirror. Expressions are difficult to gauge, as is gender or age. Due to the nature of the disorder, it is unsurprising that it can have a detrimental impact on social interaction for the individual – this may develop into social anxiety disorder or depression. In addition, they are likely to struggle with following the storyline of televised programmes. The condition can also hinder the capacity to acknowledge scenes or objects.

Without any proven treatments, research into facial recognition continues to be conducted.

Compensatory strategies are usually adopted by the individual, relying instead on other individual characteristics such as gait, hair colour or style or voice. Whilst this can work with limited success, it can be difficult to rely on, given that people may change their image or clothing frequently.

Proteus Syndrome

Incredibly rare, Proteus Syndrome is distinguished by progressive malformations and asymmetrical overgrowths of various parts of the body. Unlike most genetic conditions, Proteus syndrome is not hereditary but instead is linked with an alteration or mutation in the gene AKT1. The mutation does not affect all cells but rather a random selection, causing overgrowth in only certain body parts. It can impact bones (hyperostosis), fatty or connective tissues or blood vessels; most commonly the skulls, limbs and feet are affected. Sometimes the symptoms of Proteus syndrome can be evident from birth, characterised by certain unique facial features, but typically overgrowth does not become apparent until around 6-18 months of age at which point skeletal abnormalities tend to be the most apparent symptom.

Due to the overgrowths, there can be increased risks of atypical blood clotting, developing tumours or abnormal skin conditions. If the blood vessels have been impacted, then added complications can include deep vein thrombosis or artery blockages (pulmonary embolism).

Due to the syndrome being so rare and unique in its symptoms, treatment is approached by a multidisciplinary team of specialists to address individual symptoms. Orthopaedic specialists consider the bones and joints, dermatologists look at skin conditions, occupational therapists and physiotherapists work to improve movement whilst haematologists step in if there is a concern about blood clotting. In addition, psychosocial interventions are recommended due to the potentially difficult and isolating nature of Proteus syndrome.

Pulmonary Fibrosis

Pulmonary Fibrosis, an interstitial lung disease, is fundamentally scarring in the lungs, which can lead to breathing difficulties. Whilst rare, there are a number of known causes of pulmonary fibrosis: auto-immune (connective tissue disease-related), drug or radiation-induced, environmental (hypersensitivity pneumonitis) or occupational (pneumoconiosis). Where there is no known cause it is referred to as Idiopathic Pulmonary Fibrosis (IPF). There are also diagnoses that have been attributed to inheritable genes, though this is a small number of cases. Regardless of the cause, symptoms of pulmonary fibrosis are comparable. Breathing difficulties occur due to scarring in the lungs, which can be heard as 'crackles' when listening through a stethoscope. As such the amount of oxygen that can enter the blood is hindered so lung efficiency is reduced. In essence this can make drawing a breath that much harder, initially when doing exercise, but it can develop to impact daily activities. A persistent, hacking or dry cough, relentless fatigue and chest discomfort is also common. In some cases, clubbing may occur in the fingertips – thickened flesh under the nails causing them to curve. Poor blood circulation can also lead to other conditions such as Raynaud's syndrome.

To control or decelerate the rate of lung scarring, anti-fibrotic medicines are prescribed, whilst inflammation is reduced using steroids or immunosuppressants. Smoking antagonises the condition so support to stop is advisable. Where the cause of pulmonary fibrosis is known, for example dust or chemical allergens in the environment or a specific drug, then steps to avoid the trigger should be taken. A lung transplant may be an option for a small number of very severe cases.

Pulmonary Hypertension

The pulmonary arteries are the carriers of blood to and from the heart to the lungs; Pulmonary Hypertension (PHT) is high blood pressure, specifically in these arteries. Damage to the blood vessels means that the right-hand side of the heart (the right ventricle) has to use more exertion to move the blood into the lungs, increasing the blood pressure and eventually becoming more feeble and less efficient. Often diagnosed using a process called right heart catheterisation, there are five main types that are determined by the cause; pulmonary hypertension linked with the arteries, left heart disease, lung disease (or hypoxia, a lack of oxygen), blood clots and some other, rarer causes. It can affect people of all ages and there is an increased risk with family history of the disease.

Initial symptoms usually include feeling breathless whilst doing regular activities, combined with tiredness, a racing heartbeat and possible pain in the chest area or upper right side of the abdomen. There may also be some swelling to the legs or ankles and exercise can bring on feelings of dizziness or sometimes fainting.

The earlier the disease is identified, the better treatment can be to prevent it from causing more harm. If identifiable by another underlying cause, that will be treated in the first instance. A series of lifestyle considerations may need to be taken, particularly the implementation of a healthy, balanced diet and exercise plan, cessation of smoking and avoiding or reducing activities that can increase blood pressure, such as flying. Specific treatments are also used – anticoagulant medicines, water tablets, digoxin (to boost the heart's processes) and oxygen treatment.

Raynaud's

There are two different types of Raynaud's – primary (Raynaud's disease) which has no linked cause, and secondary (Raynaud's syndrome) which occurs due to an additional illness, usually a connective-tissue or autoimmune disorder. Both are relatively common, affecting around 5% of the UK population, though secondary Raynaud's tends to bring on more significant symptoms. The predominant trait is poor blood circulation in the bodily extremities, caused by a spasm of blood vessels.

The main symptoms include cold fingers and toes, where the skin may change colour in response to external factors of temperature or sometimes to emotional stress. Less frequently the lips, nipples, nose or earlobes can be affected. The skin typically turns pale or white, then blue as the blood vessels react, returning to a usual pink or red as the areas warm up. This process can be accompanied with pain, numbness, tingling or trouble with moving the impacted area, and may last for any time between a few minutes and a few hours.

As might be expected, the main form of treatment is to warm up the affected area to promote better circulation. Management of the condition can be improved by keeping a warm environment, wearing suitable warm clothing and practising relaxation techniques. Stimulants such as caffeine, alcohol and smoking can worsen circulation so should be done in moderation or ceased completely. A doctor may prescribe nifedipine, a medication used to improve blood circulation – depending on the severity of the condition this can be taken when required, during exposure to the cold, or daily if required.

Restless Legs Syndrome

Known also as Willis-Eknom Syndrome, Restless Legs Syndrome (RLS) is relatively common condition that results in an individual having an overpowering urge to move their legs. There is no known cause; it is believed to be linked with an iron deficiency or reduced levels of a brain neurotransmitter called dopamine. There is also evidence that the syndrome is more common in women, can run in families or can be sparked from the use of certain medications such as antihistamines, antidepressants or antipsychotics. There are two main types: primary early onset RLS (known as idiopathic) which emerges prior to the age of 45, has no specific cause and gets gradually worse, and secondary late onset RLS which appears after the age of 45 and the symptoms of which remain at a fairly consistent level.

As a spectrum condition, symptoms can range from mild to severe, with major disruption to daily life. For most people, the compulsion to move their legs is overwhelming and can be partnered with unnerving sensations running up and down the calves – fizzing, tingling, crawling, burning or throbbing. They may encounter painful cramps or a dull ache and the majority of people with RLS also experience periodic limb movements in sleep (PLMS) when the legs twitch or jolt uncontrollably a few times per minute. Lifestyle adaptations, and in particular implementing good sleep habits, are key to reducing the severity of the symptoms. Avoiding exercise, caffeine and alcohol in the evening and engaging in relaxation techniques such as gentle massage with a warm compress or having a bath can help to relieve pain and discomfort. A doctor may prescribe dopamine agonists to increase dopamine levels, sleeping aids (hypnotics) or painkillers such as codeine.

Schizophrenia

Typically emerging during early adulthood, Schizophrenia is a mental illness that affects an individual's thinking processes. There is no apparent, single cause. It has been linked to stressful life events such as bereavement, experiencing abuse, unemployment or homelessness. There is also evidence that demonstrates people with schizophrenia have a hereditary genetic predisposition or increased levels of dopamine in the brain, and there is also a strong link between the disorder and those who use cannabis or other high-potency recreational drugs.

Unlike the common misconception that people with schizophrenia have a 'split personality,' symptoms are generally categorised into positive and negative. Positive symptoms include hallucinating or having unusual, delusional beliefs. Negative symptoms, which make up the majority, tend to be loss of interest or motivation, difficulty concentrating, feelings of emotional disconnection or social avoidance and disorganised thought or speech patterns. Disrupted cognitive process can result in bad decision making, memory problems and a short attention span. Generally, the negative symptoms are less dramatic but last for a prolonged period of time, with positive ones interspersed in episodes. Dependent on the symptom emphasis, it is possible to be diagnosed with a specific type of schizophrenia – paranoid, hebephrenic, catatonic, undifferentiated, residual, simple, cenesthopathic and unspecified. Antipsychotic medication is a proved treatment for some people who have symptoms of psychosis, whereas talking-based cognitive behavioural therapy (CBT) or arts therapies can help with understanding and expression of feelings. Family intervention may be appropriate for associated relatives or carers.

Schnitzler Syndrome

Named after the dermatologist who defined it, Schnitzler or Schnitzler's Syndrome is a rare chronic autoinflammatory disease. The onset of symptoms is not characteristically seen until around the age of 55 and in line with many rare disorders, the cause remains unknown. However, many individuals have been found to have an elevated level of M-proteins in the blood, specifically one called immunoglobulin M (IgM). Known as monoclonal gammopathy, the body produces too much of the immunoglobulin and it is thought that this could be the foundation for Schnitzler syndrome.

A reddish-coloured rash not dissimilar to hives, known as urticaria, is the distinctive symptom. The rash may be raised and unlike other cases of urticaria, is not usually pruritic (itchy) in the first case, however it may become so over time. The idiosyncratic rash may only last for a few days but is likely to disappear and reappear. Typically, it is found on the torso, arms or legs and occasionally it can be exacerbated by triggers such as alcohol or stress. Fatigue, fever and pain or swelling in the bones, joints or muscles can also occur and there have been reports of enlargement of the liver, spleen and lymph nodes.

As an autoimmune disease, immunosuppressant drugs can be an effective form of treatment for Schnitzler syndrome. An interleukin-1 receptor antagonist called anakinra is the most common approach for cases where standard anti-inflammatory medication has not proven successful. Discovery and development of potential treatments continues due to the syndrome being so rare.

Scleroderma

Scleroderma, meaning "hard skin", is also described as systemic sclerosis. It is an autoimmune disease that impacts connective tissues in the body. Due to unwarranted attack from the immune system, too much collagen is produced which leads to thickening of the skin (a process known as fibrosis). There is no evidence that the condition is hereditary although there may be a genetic predisposition. Localised scleroderma and systemic scleroderma are the two different types – localised solely impacts the skin whereas systemic sclerosis is more far-reaching, concerning internal vessels and organs too.

With localised, the skin is impacted in one of two ways. Seen often in younger children, morphea is distinguishable by waxy or shiny, usually itchy, patches on the skin. Linear scleroderma, on the other hand, tends to start with a line of thickened skin which reaches deeper below the skin. Both types may get better over time, but linear sclerosis can create growth issues. Systemic sclerosis usually emerges between the ages of 30 and 50, more often in women, and affects the tissues of internal organs as well as joints and muscles. Again, there are two different types. Diffuse scleroderma can see the skin of the whole body be affected, often developing quickly. Limited cutaneous systemic scleroderma is significantly gentler and less widespread across the body, instead focused on the face, lower limbs, hands and feet.

There are a range of different treatments available given the wide variation of symptoms. Medication can be used to suppress the incorrect actions of the immune system, enhance circulation and relieve joint issues, whilst physiotherapy, massage and home-care moisturising treatments can assist in keeping skin loose and supple.

Seasonal Affective Disorder

Also referred to as 'winter depression', Seasonal Affective Disorder (SAD) is a form of depression that is directly impacted by the pattern of the seasons. Symptoms typically flare up during the winter months but tend to be less severe during the summer months. There are a number of factors that could contribute to SAD, in addition to the classic causes of depression. The amount of light that an individual is exposed to can have a direct impact on the areas of the brain that control mood; as such those who live in areas where daylight hours are altered by the seasons are potentially more likely to develop SAD. Equally, reduced daylight hours can affect the body clock, impacting sleep patterns and consequently causing depressive symptoms. Inconsistent levels of serotonin and melatonin (which affect mood and sleep) may too be responsible. It is also possible to experience symptoms during the summer months; some research has demonstrated a potential link between warmer temperatures and mental health problems.

Similar to the symptoms of depression, SAD can cause unrelenting low mood and feelings of hopelessness, worthlessness or guilt. Particular additional symptoms of SAD can include persistent tiredness or oversleeping, or an increased appetite for carbohydrates, leading to weight gain.

Given that light is believed to be a key factor in the cause of SAD, a possible form of treatment is light therapy (known as phototherapy). Artificial light is used to simulate sunlight and dawn, aiding the body's natural sleep/wake cycle. Talking therapies and antidepressant medication can also be recommended forms of treatment.

Sjögren's Syndrome

The long-term autoimmune condition Sjögren's Syndrome impacts the whole body but is most renowned for symptoms that cause widespread dryness in the eyes and mouth. Substantially more present in women than men, the condition usually emerges between the ages of 45 and 60 and in around half of diagnoses it is cited as a direct complication of an additional autoimmune disease (mostly lupus or rheumatoid arthritis).

Predominantly the glands responsible for producing tears and saliva are involved. Dry eyes may be itchy, red, swollen or painful and can also be accompanied with double vision. A dry mouth can cause extreme thirst, impact eating and swallowing, cause voice alterations and lead to further issues such as mouth ulcers or gingivitis (gum disease). Dryness may also spread to other areas of the body, resulting in dry skin or rashes, a dry, persistent cough, vaginal dryness in women and join pain or stiffness. Internally it can also cause malfunction of the kidneys, lungs, liver or other organs and it may increase an individual's chance of developing lymphoma.

Treatments are aimed at reducing dryness in the affected areas. For eyes, various over-the-counter eye drops may be suitable for minor symptoms. For more persistent or severe cases, anti-inflammatory eye drops, such as cyclosporin, might be prescribed, or a medication named pilocarpine which encourages production of fluid, might be prescribed. Good oral hygiene, reducing the intake of alcohol or certain foods and stopping smoking can help to reduce mouth dryness and a range of possible saliva substitutes can be recommended by a pharmacist.

Sleep Disorders

Sleep Disorders are varied in their impact, typically affecting an individual's ability to obtain and maintain healthy, consistent sleep. Over 100 individual sleep disorders have been identified, some of which are severely detrimental to an individual's daily functioning. They can generally be classified into six different categories – insomnias, hypersomnolence disorders, sleep movement disorders, parasomnias, sleep-related breathing disorders and circadian rhythm sleep-wake disorders. The most eminent disorder is insomnia, which to some extent is thought to affect just under a third of all adults. Insomnia is broadly the complexity of falling asleep or staying asleep, which is problematic for around three months or longer. Hypersomnolence disorders, or hypersomnias, are characterised by feelings of overwhelming fatigue and sleepiness during the day, such as narcolepsy. If a person experiences abnormal movement during a period of sleep, such as restless legs syndrome or bruxism (teeth grinding) then this can be considered a sleep-related disorder. Parasomnias include sleepwalking, night terrors and REM (rapid-eye movement) sleep behaviour disorder. As the name suggests, sleep-related breathing disorders cause disruption to inhalation and exhalation. Sleep apnoea is the most prevalent, physiological factor which results in pauses in breathing during sleep. Sleep-wake disorders impact circadian rhythms, the internal body clock – these can be triggered by shift work or jet lag.

Treatments are varied depending on the condition. Practicing good sleep hygiene is key, avoiding alcohol or caffeine, turning off electronic screens, practicing relaxation and adopting a bedtime routine. Sleeping pills or supplements can be used as well as specific breathing devices, dental guards or surgery.

Spinal Muscular Atrophy

There are a number of different types of the neuromuscular disorder Spinal Muscular Atrophy (SMA), categorised by the age at which the symptoms first emerge. All types are caused by a defective gene (SMN1) passed down from both parents, although in some rare cases it can be inherited from just one parent. SMN1 determines a protein which is responsible for motor neurons; the loss of these are the cause of the symptoms associated with the condition: muscle wastage (atrophy) which precedes weakness and motion loss. Type 0 is present in the foetus, whilst type 1 is the most common and is diagnosed before the age of 6 months. Babies will have severely weak muscle tone (hypotonia) and due to consequent breathing and eating complications, often will not survive beyond a few years. Type 2 is found in babies ages 7 – 18 months and will also present weak muscles but are generally able to hold themselves up in the seated position. Respiratory muscle strength is typically weak, leading to an increased probability of chest infections, and scoliosis (curvature of the spine) is relatively commonplace. Life expectancy may be shortened but not for the majority. Type 3 is diagnosed after the age of 18 months until late childhood and causes balance or walking problems, whilst type 4 (or adult-onset SMA) may develop into walking difficulties over time. Weak and shaking or trembling muscles can be associated with all types. Treatment priorities depend on individual symptoms and age. For young babies they will likely need breathing and feeding assistance, whilst older children and adults require a focus on assistive equipment, physiotherapy and potential surgery to address the issue of scoliosis.

Syringomyelia

Syringomyelia is the growth of a cyst filled with fluid, known as a syrinx, located within the spinal cord. Whilst there a few possible causes, the bulk of cases are the result of a brain defect called Chiari malformation, when there is a protrusion of tissue in the brain into the spinal canal at the craniovertebral junction. As such the condition is sometimes referred to as congenital syringomyelia. Disease or injury to the spinal cord and meningitis have also been linked as causes. If there is no known cause, it is classified as primary syringomyelia.

Subject to the location of the syrinx, some individuals may have the condition but be asymptomatic, showing no noticeable signs. Others may experience a slow progression of symptoms, typically gradual muscle wastage, stiffness or pain in the back, shoulders and neck area. Reflex speed may be reduced and sensitivity to temperature can be decreased. Some people develop a curvature of the spine (scoliosis) and in the worst cases the arms and legs can end up paralysed.

For those who are asymptomatic or if the condition has little impact on the individual, there is no need to intervene with treatment, providing it is monitored. Physical therapy can improve muscle strength as well as motion, balance and stability. Surgery is the usual method of treatment for serious cases – removal of bone from the skull to relieve pressure, correcting a malformation such as a tethered spinal cord or bony growth, or using a shunt to drain the syrinx of fluid.

Tardive Dyskinesia

A rare condition depicted by involuntary, spontaneous movements of the face or body, Tardive Dyskinesia (TD) is commonly associated with and a possible side effect of antipsychotic medication taken in the treatment of mental disorders. Not everyone who takes dopamine receptor blockers develops the condition and it is not clear why; long-term usage is believed to be responsible for generating brain biochemical abnormalities which is cited as a possible origin. TD is a neurological movement disorder which causes jerky, uncontrollable actions such as poking out the tongue, smacking lips, repeated blinking or grimacing of the face. Beyond the facial area it can trigger movement in the hands or feet, which may be quick or slow, writhing or twisted. If symptoms develop in a relatively short period of time or the muscles spasm greatly, it can be an indication of the more serious tardive dystonia.

Early awareness of the symptoms is key – there is no assurance that the symptoms will ease when medication is stopped, though they may reduce in severity over time. On the contrary, coming off the medication may also cause new symptoms or worsen existing ones. As TD can be emotionally challenging, an emphasis on mental and physical wellbeing is paramount for dealing with the condition on a day-to-day basis. There are various medications, typically used to treat epilepsy or Huntingdon's disease, as well as some herbal supplements or remedies that may prove helpful in reducing movements. For some, massage is beneficial for easing muscular pain.

Temporomandibular Joint Disorder

The temporomandibular joint is the hinge that permits movement of the jaw, connecting it to the skull's temporal bones. Temporomandibular Joint Disorder (TMD) is indicated when there is pain or limited movement in this area. There are several possible causes of TMD. A previous jaw or muscular injury, particularly whiplash, or arthritis within the joint can lead to symptoms. Similarly, intense clenching or grinding of the teeth can do it, regularly brought on by stress.

The pain caused by TMD can be severe – it might start in the jaw area but can spread to other areas of the face, ears, neck or upper shoulders. It can prevent the mouth from being opened particularly wide or the jaw can seemingly get locked into place when either open or closed. Some people may experience sounds akin to a pop or click when moving the jaw whilst others may feel like their bite and teeth are misaligned. Further added complications can be headaches, earaches or toothache.

Taking pharmacy-recommended anti-inflammatory painkillers is often the first step to relieving the symptoms. Pressing a hot or cold compress over the painful jaw area, keeping to a diet of soft foods and utilising relaxation techniques can largely help too. If the problem negatively impacts sleeping, a dentist might prescribe stronger painkillers or muscle relaxants. They may also suggest a night guard or splint to be worn over the teeth to prevent grinding. For the most acute cases, additional treatments can include tigger-point injections, radio wave therapy, low-level laser therapy or at times surgical procedures.

Tourette's Syndrome

Typically emerging during childhood or adolescence, Tourette's Syndrome is characterised by uncontrolled sounds and movements, known as tics. It is thought to affect around 1% of children, impacting more boys than girls, with most initial symptoms developing around the ages of 5 to 7 years old. Many children also have associated conditions of obsessive compulsive disorder (OCD), anxiety or attention deficit hyperactive disorder (ADHD). Beyond the evident neurological dysfunction, it is not understood what causes Tourette's although it is thought that an imbalance of the brain chemical dopamine could be responsible. There is proof that tics run in families and environmental factors such as anxiety or stress can be seen to aggravate them.

Tics are classified as either motor (movement related) or phonic (vocal). Examples of motor tics include jerking movements, facial movements and eye rolling or blinking. Phonic tics include whistling, sniffing, clicking the tongue or sometimes making animal noises. Contrary to popular belief, only around 10% of individuals display symptoms of involuntary swearing (clinically known as coprolalia). As tics are preceded with an unvoluntary urge, some people are able to temporarily suppress the tic. For many children, estimated at approximately half of all cases, the symptoms will have noticeably decreased by the time they reach adulthood.

There is no cure for Tourette's. Habit reversal training and exposure with response prevention (ERP) have both shown to be effective forms of behavioural therapy to help the individual train and control their tics. Medication is also an option but not particularly commonplace.

Transverse Myelitis

Transverse Myelitis is a rare neurological disorder that causes damage to the myelin, the defensive substance that surrounds fibres in the nerve cells. As an infection is seen to precede onset of the disorder in around half of all cases, transverse myelitis is believed to be an autoimmune condition that causes inflammation to the spinal cord. It can also be linked to other conditions such as multiple sclerosis, lupus and some cancers or vascular disorders. Unlike many other disorders there is no evidence of genetic influence. Cases tend to lean towards a slight majority of women and the two peak age groups for a diagnosis are 10 to 19 and 30 to 39, although it can affect people of any age group.

Symptoms of the disorder tend to develop quite rapidly, from a few hours to a few weeks, and there are four main aspects: pain in the lower back or legs, weakness in the either one of both legs or arm muscles, unusual sensations (known as paresthesia) similar to prickling, burning or tickling in the legs, and complications with the bowel or bladder. Partial or full paralysis of the legs can occur in intense cases. Treatment is seen to have varying degrees of success; some people are able to make a full recovery whereas others can end up with a permanent disability. Medication is used for pain relief whilst neuro-focused physiotherapy aims to improve issues with balance and mobility. Oral or intravenous corticosteroids are used to lower swelling and is often enhanced with plasmapheresis (plasma exchange therapy) to limit further damage by the immune system.

Trigeminal Neuralgia

The trigeminal nerve is located within the skull and is responsible for touch and pain sensations in the face, as well as controlling the muscles used for chewing and biting. Sometimes referred to as tic douloureux, Trigeminal Neuralgia is characterised by severe but short bouts of pain in the jaw area. More likely to be diagnosed over the age of 50, primary trigeminal neuralgia is caused by irritation or compression of the nerve from a blood vessel pressing on the area. Sometimes it is due to an impairment of the protective myelin sheath layer around the trigeminal nerve – called secondary trigeminal neuralgia, instigated by injury, trauma, or an additional condition such as multiple sclerosis. There is a trigeminal nerve running down both sides of the face; usually pain is only felt on one side but in some rare cases it can be both. The jaw, teeth and lower section of the face are usually the most affected, but it can be known to spread to the forehead area too. Type 1 (classic) is distinguished by periods of unexpected stabbing pain that come and go in remission, whereas type 2 (atypical) is a constant throbbing, dull ache. Simple everyday activities such as brushing teeth, drinking, smiling or talking can act as triggers. It can take its toll on emotional wellbeing and lead to additional psychological conditions.

As a form of nerve pain, trigeminal neuralgia is typically treated with anticonvulsants, specifically one called carbamazepine. As its effectiveness may dwindle over time, surgery may become an alternative. There are a few options: percutaneous procedures, stereotactic radiosurgery or microvascular decompression.

Ulcerative Colitis

Ulcerative Colitis is a chronic condition and form of Inflammatory Bowel Disease (IBD), along with Crohn's Disease. It impacts the large intestine (colon) and the rectum, resulting in swelling and ulceration (the development of ulcers) of the inner lining. This affects the body's ability to process waste, typically causing abdominal issues and recurrent bowel movements. There is no evident cause of ulcerative colitis – medics believe it is a combination of problems with the immune system, genetic factors and various environmental triggers. Depending on the area of the bowel that is affected, the condition is categorised into three types, each one with more typical symptoms. In proctitis, the rectum is the only inflamed area, resulting in rectal pain or bleeding and an increased need for bowel movements. Left-sided colitis affects the rectum and descending colon area, associated with bouts of mucus or blood-filled diarrhoea and abdominal pain on the left-hand side. Pancolitis, or total colitis, correlates to the whole colon and sees an increase in the severity and range of symptoms – frequent diarrhoea, sometimes interspersed with mucus or pus, and pain across the abdominal area. It can also cause a loss of appetite leading to weight loss, as well as iron deficiency anaemia and problems outside the gut chiefly in the joints, skin, eyes and liver.

Drugs to target and ease inflammation of the intestine lining called aminosalicylates (5-ASAs) can be taken either taken long-term or when a flare up of symptoms occurs. Corticosteroids, immunosuppressants and biological drugs may also be prescribed. If the condition is detrimental to daily living, a surgical procedure called a colectomy to remove the colon can be considered.

Vascular Dementia

After Alzheimer's disease, Vascular Dementia is the leading cause of dementia - a syndrome, rather than a disease, related to the decline in a brain's normal level of functioning. A vascular dementia diagnosis is rare under the age of 65 and symptoms tend to develop and get worse over time. It is caused by a reduction in blood circulation to the brain, often due to the blood vessels narrowing, a process known as subcortical vascular dementia. It can also happen as a result of a stroke (single-infarct dementia) or a series of small strokes and blood clots called transient ischaemic attacks (multi-infarct dementia). The impact of the condition is primarily seen in mental ability, with earlier symptoms including difficulty understanding, concentrating, and planning. Depending on which part of the brain has been affected, thought processes may slow down and there can be some issues with memory. As the symptoms worsen, either gradually or in swifter steps of succession, there may be signs of disorientation, loss of balance or bladder control and noticeable changes in personality.

Treatment is sometimes successful for slowing down the progression of the condition and preventing any additional damage to the brain. A comprehensive care plan is made with the aim of targeting the individual underlying cause. Lifestyle changes to diet, alcohol consumption, smoking and daily exercise are usually advised. Medication is used to treat high blood pressure, high cholesterol or reducing the risk of additional blood clots and strokes (anticoagulant medicines). Dementia-specific activities that have also been found to improve mental wellbeing, from dementia cafes, reminiscence work, arts-based activities and singing.

SUMMARY

For so many people living with illnesses and disabilities, their condition goes unnoticed and is invisible to those around them. Much is still unknown about the causes of numerous conditions and with many having similar overlapping or subjective symptoms, the journey to an accurate diagnosis can be lengthy and frustrating. With a blend of genetics and biological, social and environmental factors involved, sometimes in partnership with a secondary condition, knowing the cause can be the first step to managing the illness. Though some conditions are treatable, many are not. From chronic illnesses, diabetes or arthritis, to sleep or anxiety disorders and other mental health conditions, living with an invisible illness can be incredibly isolating and debilitating. Daily life can feel like a battle against pain, discomfort or limitations that impact the ability to work, socialise or live comfortably at home. Sharing the reality of living with an invisible illness with family, friends and colleagues can help to reduce the potential misunderstanding and perceived stigma around it. For some conditions, particularly the rarer ones, it can be challenging to find or access support or assistance. Many health charities provide a host of information, whilst their online or in-person communities offer a support network to bring together those with shared experiences of the condition. Millions of people are currently living with invisible illnesses – none of them are alone.

www.ingramcontent.com/pod-product-compliance
Lightning Source LLC
Chambersburg PA
CBHW070630220526
45466CB00001B/143